# A Life *with* Alzheimer's

## Caregiver's Workbook

*The Caregiver's Guide along
with additional pages
for reflection and action.*

## FROM

## *A to Z*

## By Verna R. Jacobs

**A Life with ALZ**
A Life with Alzheimer's: Caregiver's Workbook

**Edition**
Copyright by © 2017 Verna R. Jacobs

**ISBN**
ISBN-13: 978-1977754486
ISBN-10: 1977754481

Printed in the United States of America

Photography, Editing by
MeShayle Lester

Published by
Kingdom Reach Technologies, LLC.
P. O. Box 165882
Irving, Texas 75016
(214) 774-4731

# Caregiving Tips

This book include tips that have
helped me care for my dad.

**May you find this information beneficial
to you and your loved one.**

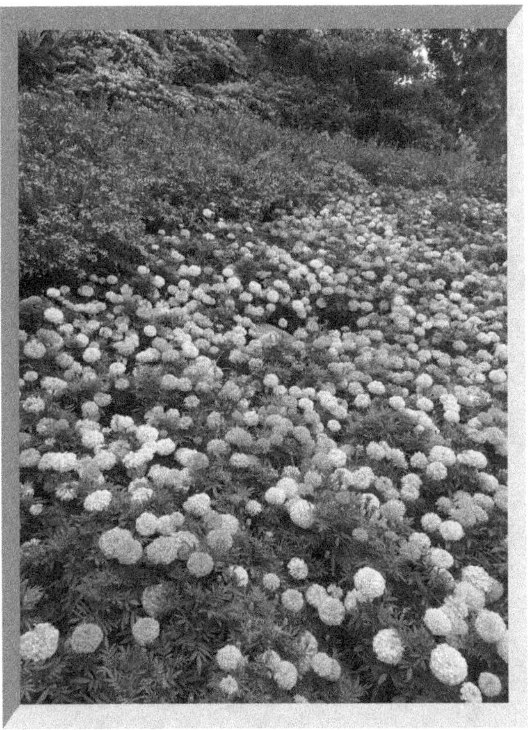

Additional resources can be found in the
Reference section or online at alifewithalz.com.

# Accept / New Norm

Accept the new norm.  Stop expecting what used to be.

Dad had to accept his limitations and he also had to accept that things were changing beyond his control.

Me, in response to Dad wanting to drive: "Remember when the sheriff pulled you over for driving erratically?  I'll be your chauffeur, so you don't have to worry about driving.  Let's go in my car."

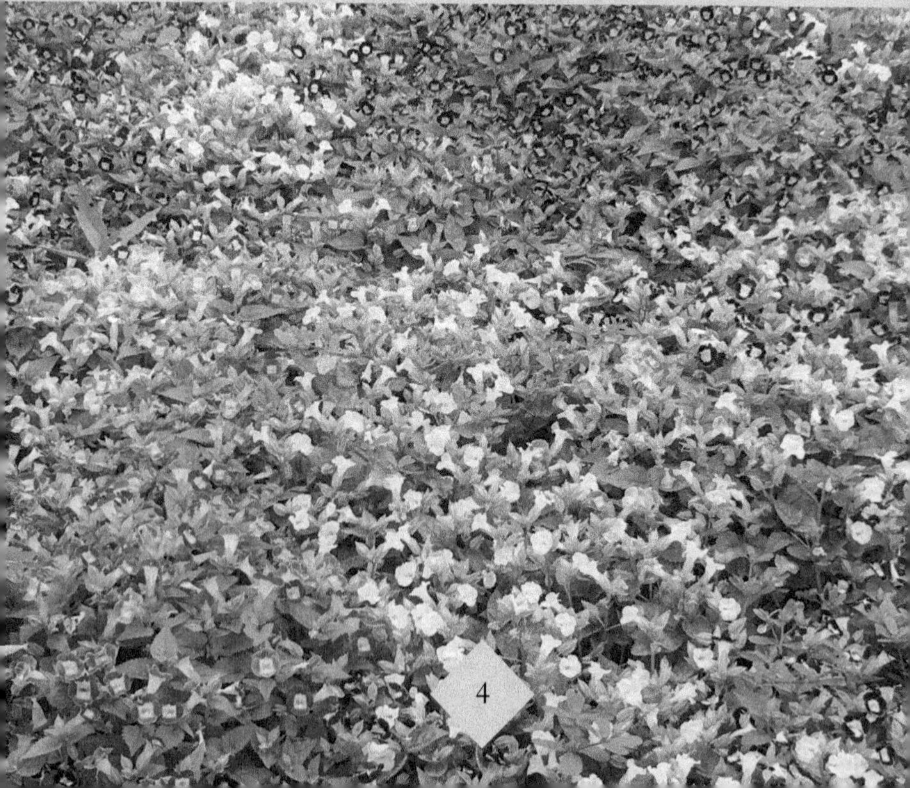

# Reflection / Action:

*What are some of the new norms for your loved one? How can you respond to these new norms to make the transition easier?*

# Accusations

Accusations can be a result of unresolved conflicts or unexpressed emotions.

Here are two examples of an exchange I had with dad:

> **Dad:** "Why are you looking at me that way?"
> **Me:** "I apologize for looking at you that way."

> **Dad:** "Someone was in the house and took my wallet"
> **Me:** "No one has been here. Let me help you find it."

We once found his wallet under the mattress and another time we found it in the shirt drawer.  When I kept helping him find his missing wallet and acknowledged the importance of helping him do so, this behavior stopped.  He knew that I was on his side, and that I was there to help.

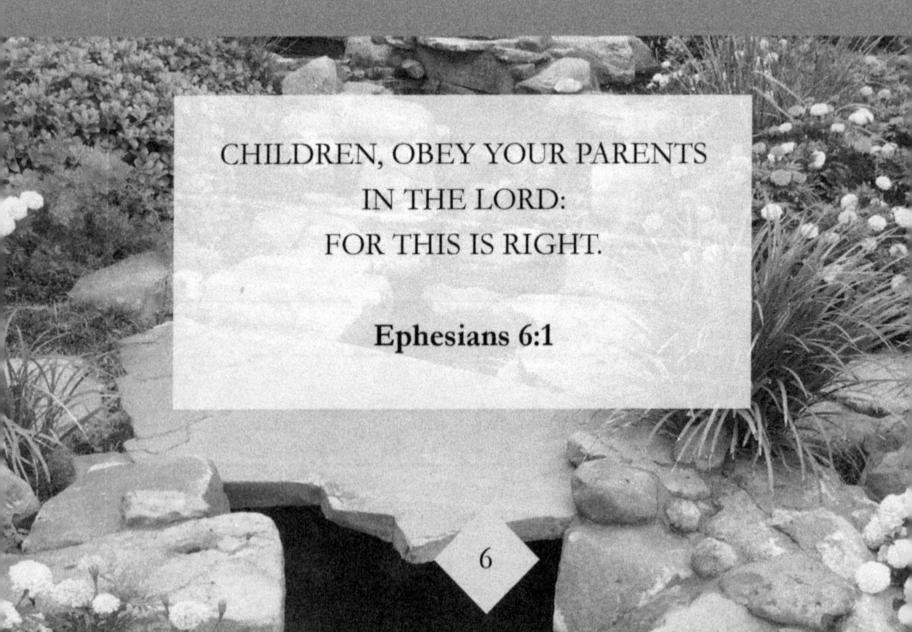

# Reflection | Action:

*Note any unresolved conflicts or unexpressed emotions regarding your loved one. Consider ways to respond respectively to these emotions in order to build trust.*

# Affirmation

Sincere affirmation and recognition of one's contribution is a basic need.

After the yardman leaves or dad comes inside from picking up leaves from the driveway, a compliment is in order for the great job he does in keeping the yard looking nice. That warrants dad getting up, looking out the window or going outside to confirm a job well done.

When he completes his word finds puzzles, this is another opportunity for me to acknowledge his eye for detail and ease in finding all the words.

Look for moments to affirm!

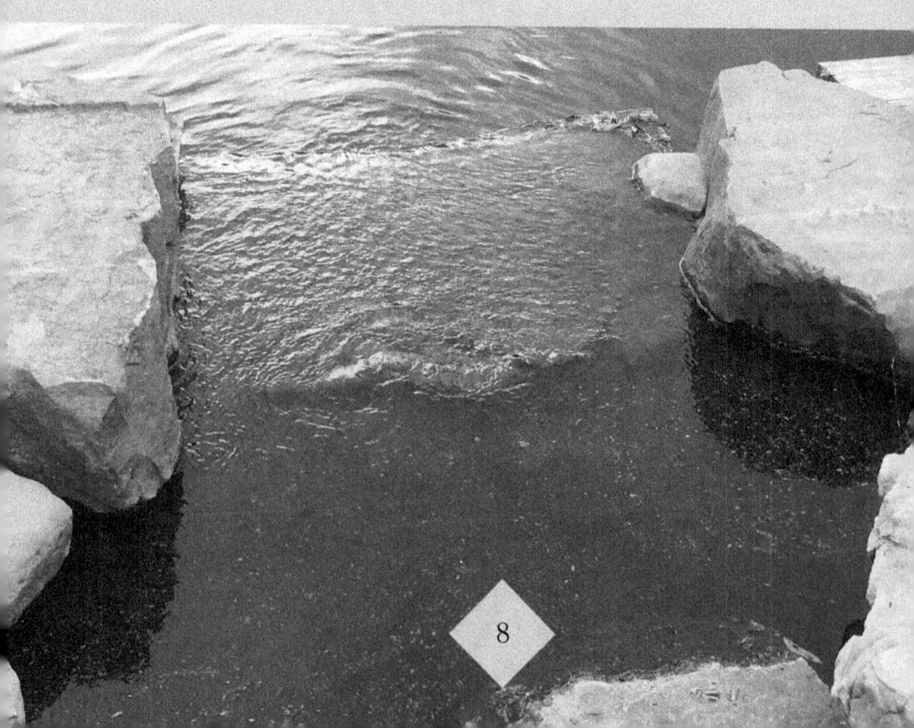

# Reflection / Action:

*Record moments that might serve as an opportunity to acknowledge and affirm your loved one for a job well done?*

# Be Prepared / Remember the Scouts

It never ceases to amaze me how people with children seem unprepared when taking them out in public, especially if there might be wait time. As a former Girl Scout, I remember one should always be prepared.

Likewise, when taking your loved one to the doctor's office, store or just riding in the car, an elder bag is in order. It should include Kleenex, bottled water, snacks, sun shades, cap, extra jacket, busy work, i.e. word finds, magazine and paper/pen. In addition, a change of clothes should be in the trunk of the car. This helps adjust to different environments and prepares you for the unexpected.

Grab a buggy for them to hold on to when shopping or grab a wheel chair, if one is accessible.

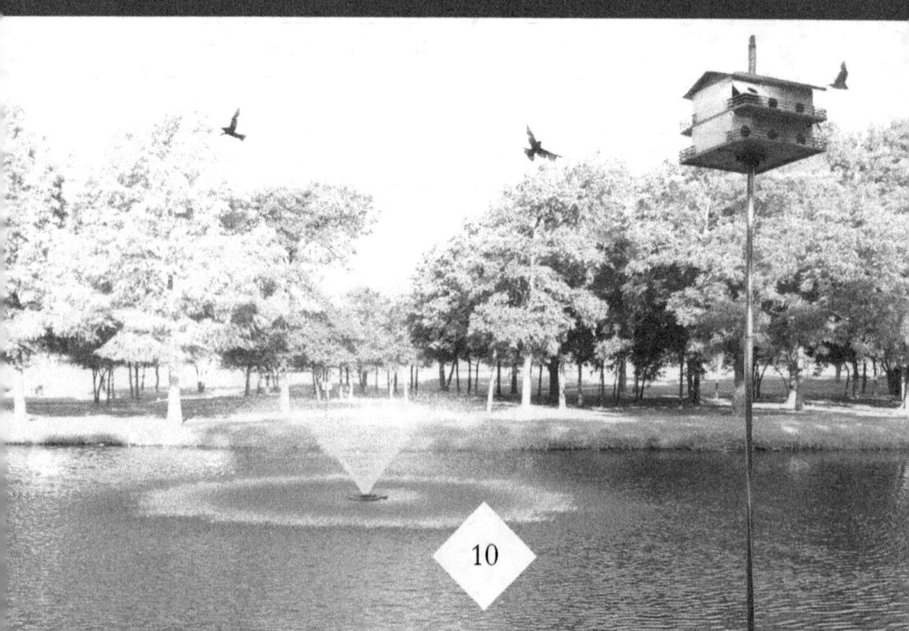

# Reflection / Action:

*List some of the items your loved one can't leave home without.*

# Become / Believe

Become what is needed.  Stop looking elsewhere for what you can provide.  Reduce the stress.

I learned to clip dad's hair, shave him and give him a sponge bath.  This took time, trust and patience.

Learning what is not effective, helps to learn what works.

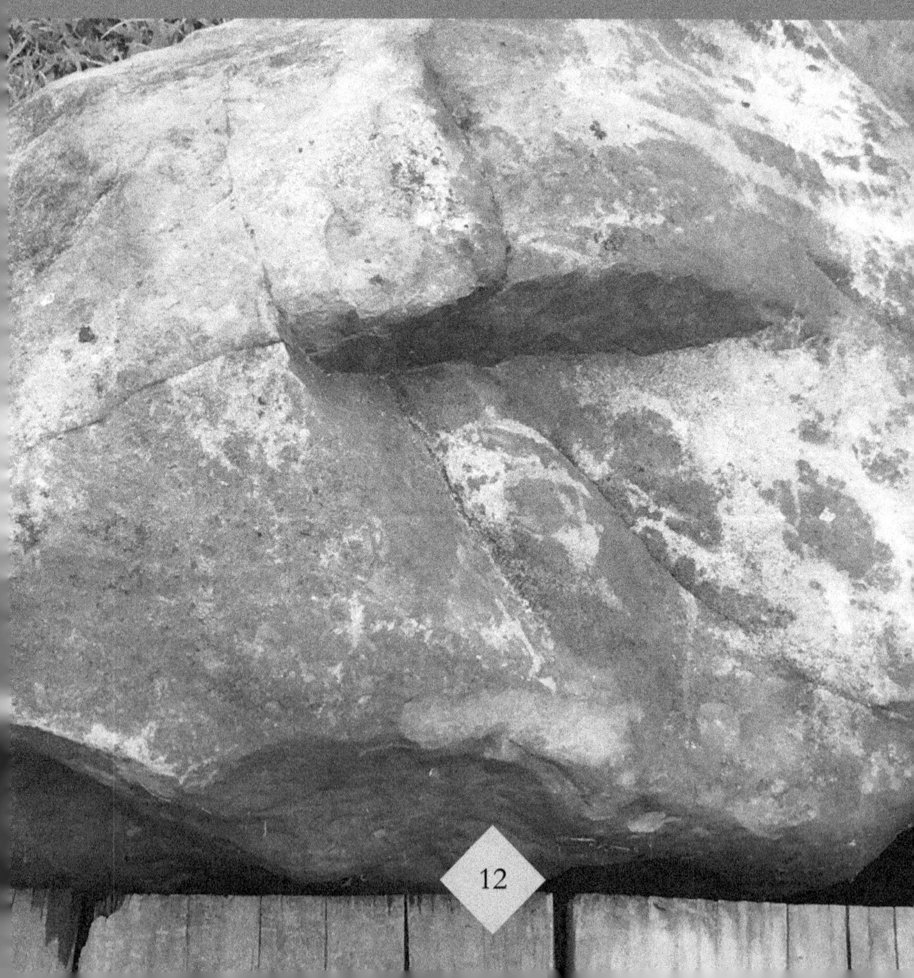

<h1 align="center">*Reflection / Action:*</h1>

13

*What are some of the services you can provide to help reduce stress for you and your loved one?  List things that are not effective that you may need support with?*

____________________________________________________

____________________________________________________

____________________________________________________

____________________________________________________

____________________________________________________

____________________________________________________

____________________________________________________

____________________________________________________

____________________________________________________

____________________________________________________

____________________________________________________

____________________________________________________

# Care

Show care and concern.  Extend care.  It only takes a few more seconds to do.  For example: A tuck, a prayer and a kiss when time for bed.

**Me:**  "I'll be over here if you need me."
**Dad:**  "I'll be right here if you need me."

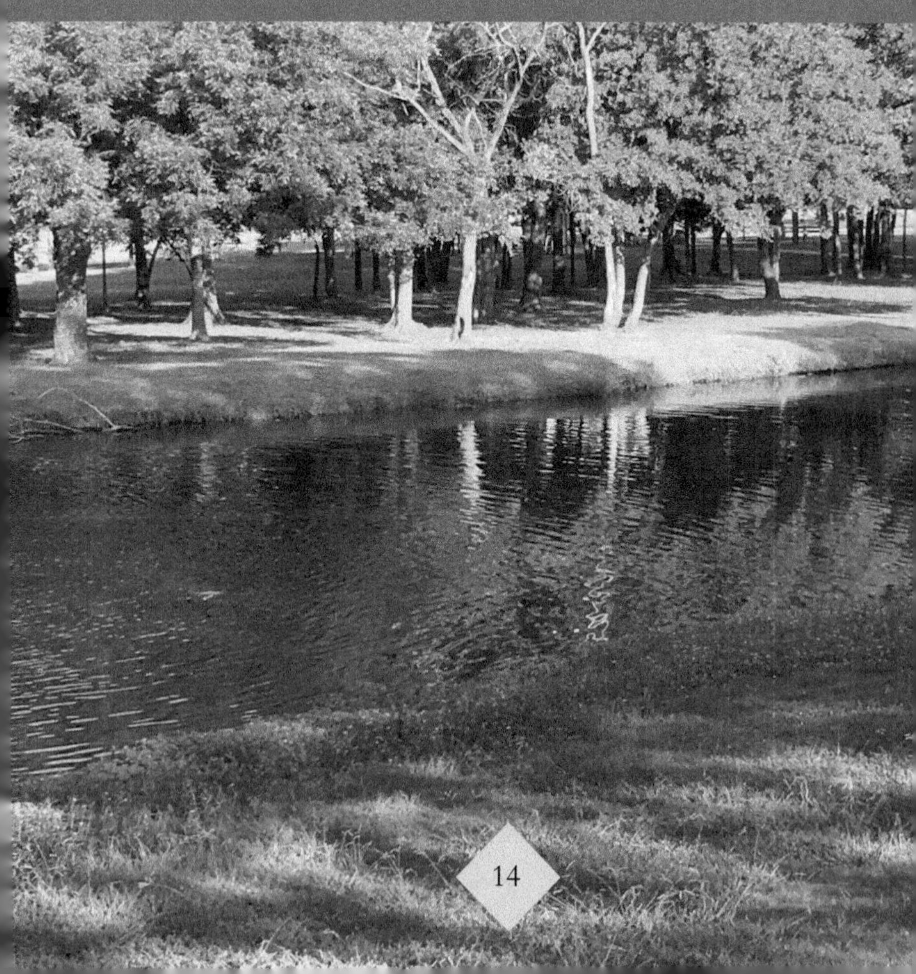

# Reflection / Action:

*Record things that can be done to show care and concern.*

# Caregiver Frustration – Rehab Facility

*Be aware of some of the frustrations that can incur as a result to healthcare facilities:*

- Limited options regarding facilities for persons with Alzheimer's.

- Skilled care facility with limited staff, different staff each shift rotation, inconsistent protocol, inconsistent daily regiments and personal hygiene care, minimum physical and occupational therapy and lack of security.

- Professionals who disregard patient privacy rights and discuss matters in front of other patients and professionals who do not need to know.

- Inaccurate documentation or emotionally written nurse's notes and care plan.

- **Dad's response to these frustrations:** "Much to do about nothing!"

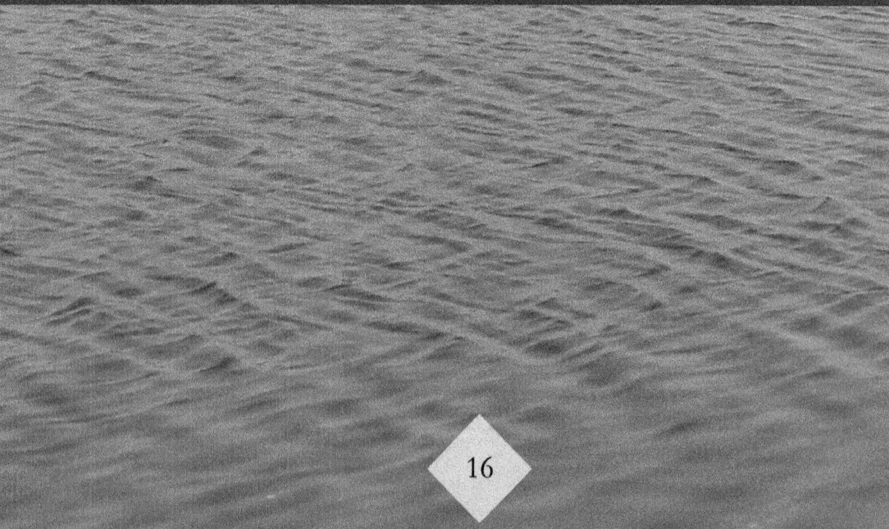

# Reflection / Action:

*Note any frustrations that you might have.*

# Declutter

*Decluttering gives a sense of order and refreshing.*

» Get rid of old newspapers, magazines and junk mail.

» Give away clothes too small, too big, worn or obsolete. This is necessary.

» Declutter walkways, i.e. hallways and pathways to common areas. Removing excess furniture is safety prevention.

» Throw away expired prescription medications, over-the-counter medications, foods and house products is paramount.

# Reflection / Action:

*List ways you can declutter your living space.*

# Different Levels of Care

*During an extended stay at the hospital, one can observe different kind of health care staff:*

**Loud and Insensitive** – They come in the door talking loud, cracking jokes and hollering to friends down the hall. Then, they want to ask the sick patient why they are not jovial.

**Surface Workers** – They don't call you by name but a pet name. Some do just enough to get by.  They don't update the board with their name or care about input and out take of fluids.  Performance may not be by protocol.  They only check certain things when asked to do so.

**Attentive but Legalistic** – They are attentive to the family, but very legalistic and opinionated.  If one has a broken hip and dementia, why would you ask the patient the level of pain from 1-10 each time you give the scheduled meds.  Pain is Pain, so just give the meds.

**Professional** – They love what they do and are sensitive to people and thorough in their job.  They are attentive to what the patient and family concerns are and always give an extra level of care.

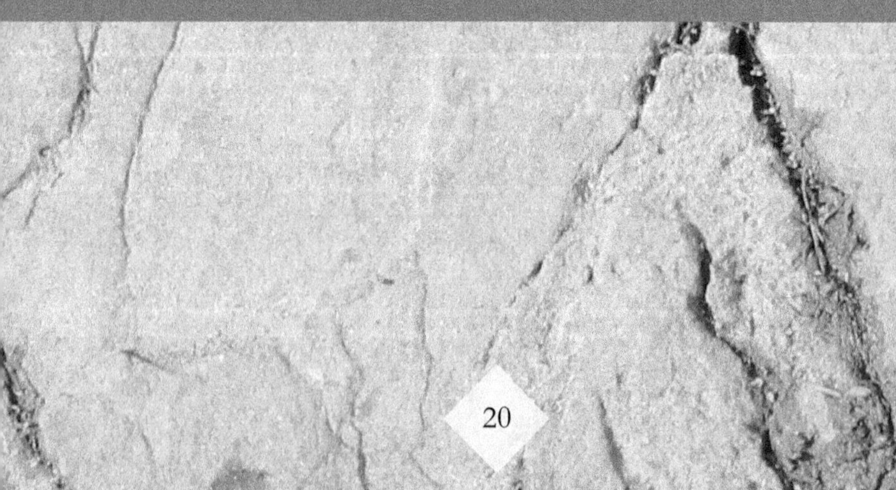

# Dignity

Our loved ones should never be forced to do something they do not want to do, when they can vocalize their opinion.

When it comes to personal care, sometimes we have to be creative in the approach. Advising that someone is coming by today or that we have a doctor's appointment can get the ball rolling.

Sometimes they are aware it is time to freshen up and welcome the assistance, especially when it takes a long time to do tasks that were once easy.  Other times, you go with the flow!  Maintaining their dignity is more important sometimes.

Being inclusive when talking to healthcare workers or other when dealing with their affairs helps them feel a part of the process. Always speak in a positive manner, not condescending, but vocalize your observations and obtain clarity if a change needs to be made.

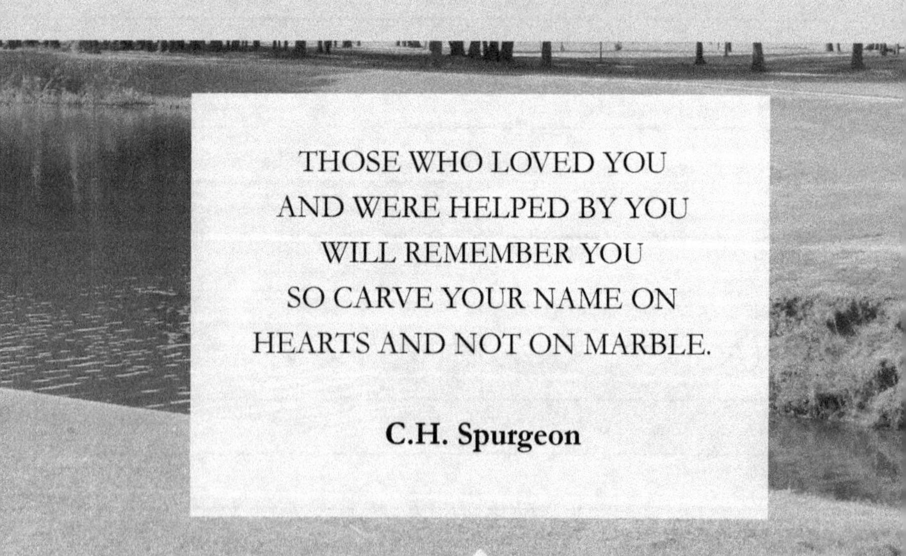

# Reflection / Action:

*Consider ways you can show dignity to your loved one and show inclusion.*

# Does He Need That?

After careful observation, review of drug side effects and interactions, and journaling of loved one's behavior changes, I asked for a review of drugs and over-the-counter medications.

## *It's time for a review when:*

- They seem drugged and are not functional.

- Their blood pressure drops too quickly and they have to go lie down.

- You are noticing usual side effects.

- Meds are not doing what the doctor says it is to treat.

- Different drugs are for the same thing or perhaps prescribed by different doctors or specialists.

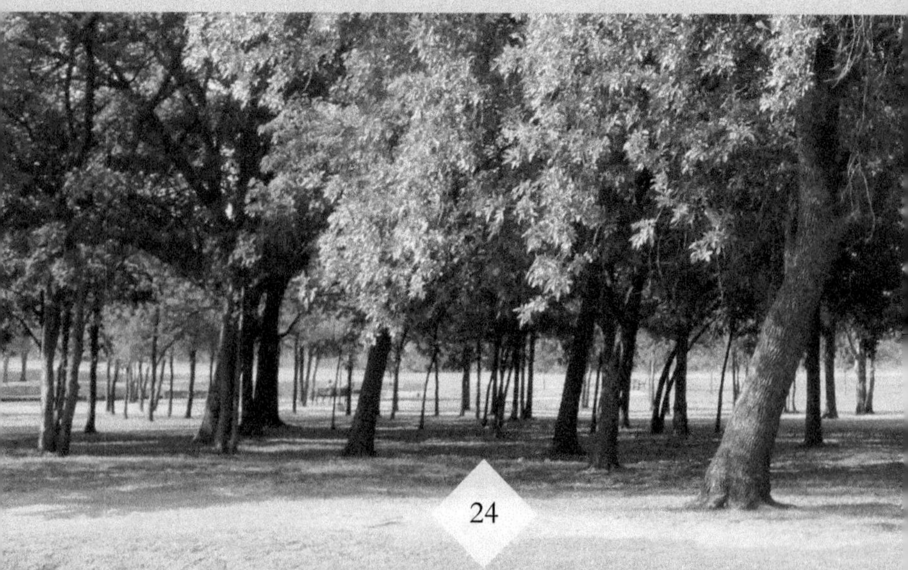

<h1 align="center">Reflection | Action:</h1>

*Make a list of medications prescribed and their common side effects.*

# Don't Quit / Like Retail

If you have ever worked the floor in a retail store, you know the work never ends when keeping the racks and shelves nice and neat. It can be accomplished if you don't have customers.

Caring for someone with incontinence is just like working retail. When you get your loved one freshened up and changed; bed, floors and carpet cleaned; and clothes washed; then you can sit down and relax.

Is there a sense of accomplishment if you are back to square one? Working the floor in retail, is more about appearances and maintenance, than productivity.

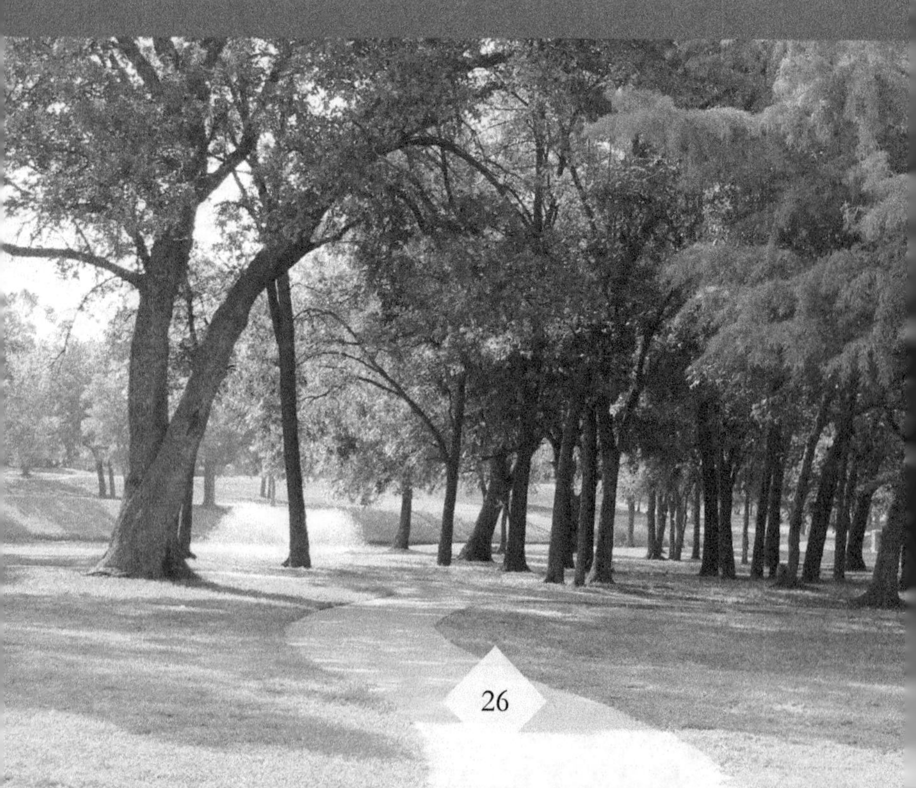

# Eye Level

Make sure every thing needed by your loved one is visible and at eye level.  Daily and commonly used items such as frequently read books, toiletries (toothbrush, comb, deodorant), underwear, snacks, kitchen utensils should be accessible.

Likewise, items that may be harmful such as sharp objects, medicines, and cleaning fuilds should be out of sight.

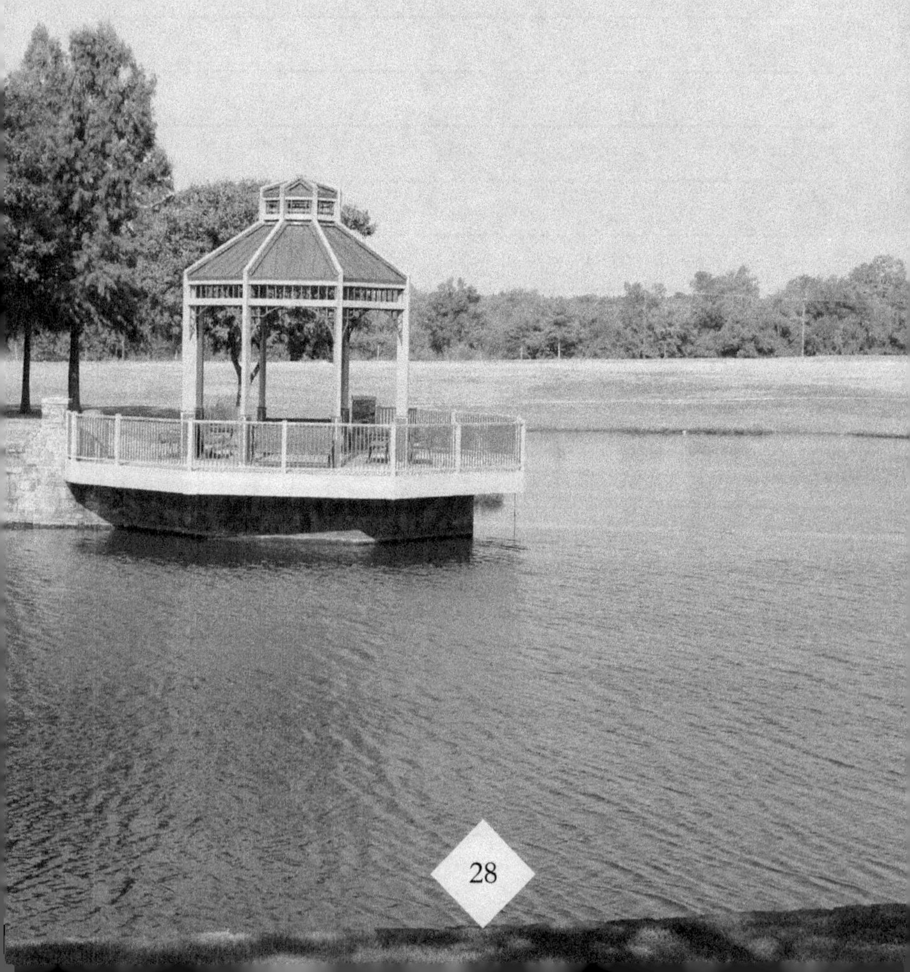

# Reflection | Action:

*What are some commonly used items that need to be more accessible?*

# Evaluate

Evaluate and re-evaluate if medications and procedures are necessary.  Do your own research.  Contact health provider to ensure coverage and in-network providers save money.  Check the effectiveness and side effectives of prescriptions and over the counter (OTC) medications.

Evaluate home services and monthly bills.  What is contractual?  Are you getting the best rates?

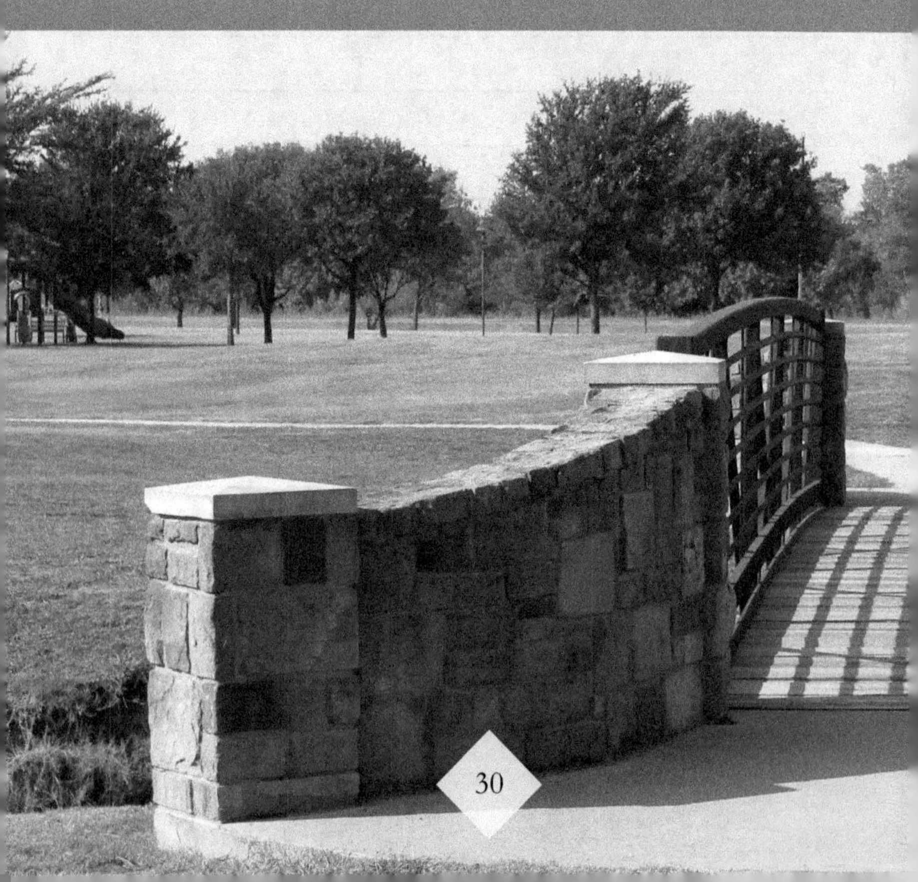

## Reflection / Action:

*Make a list of services that need to be evaluated.*

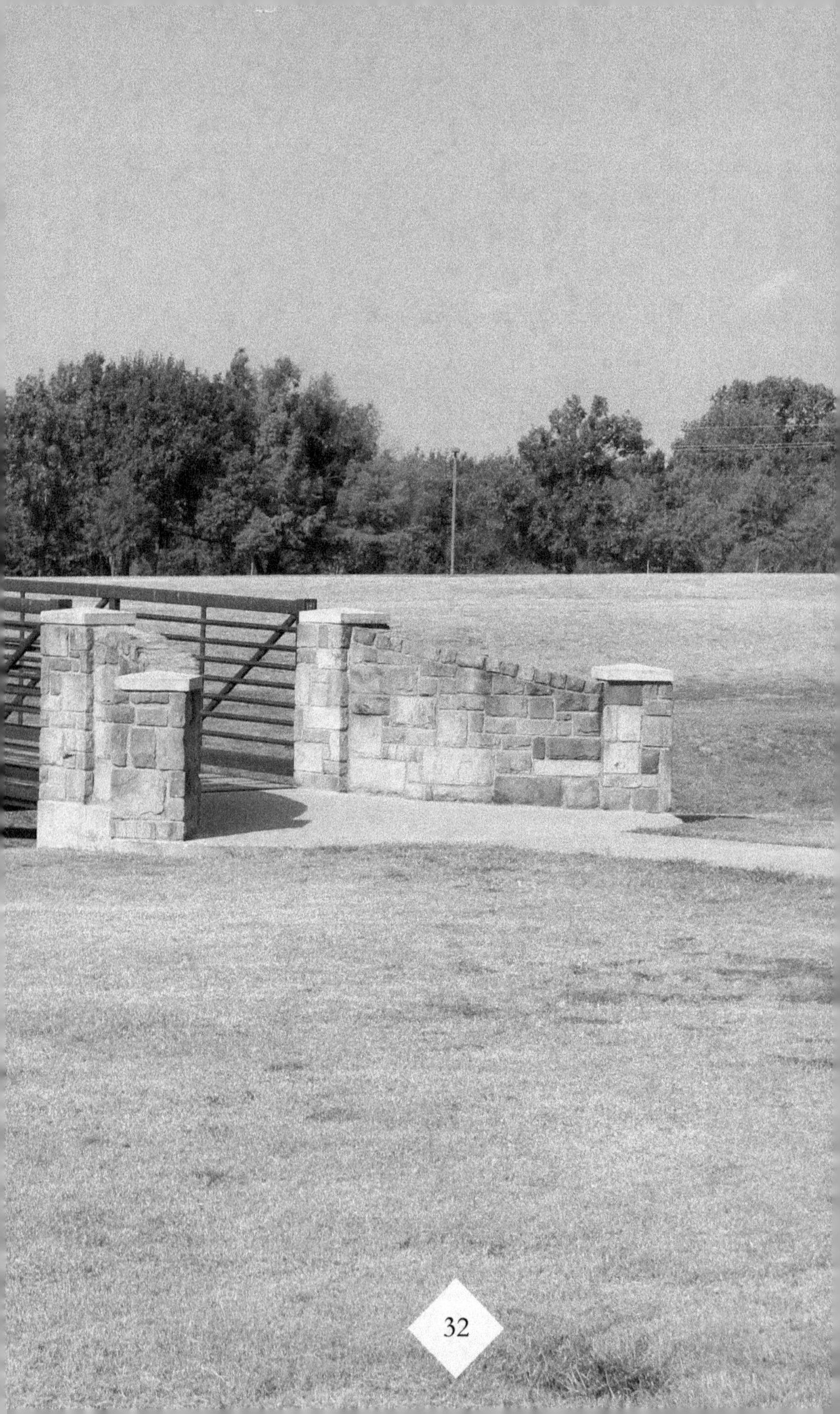

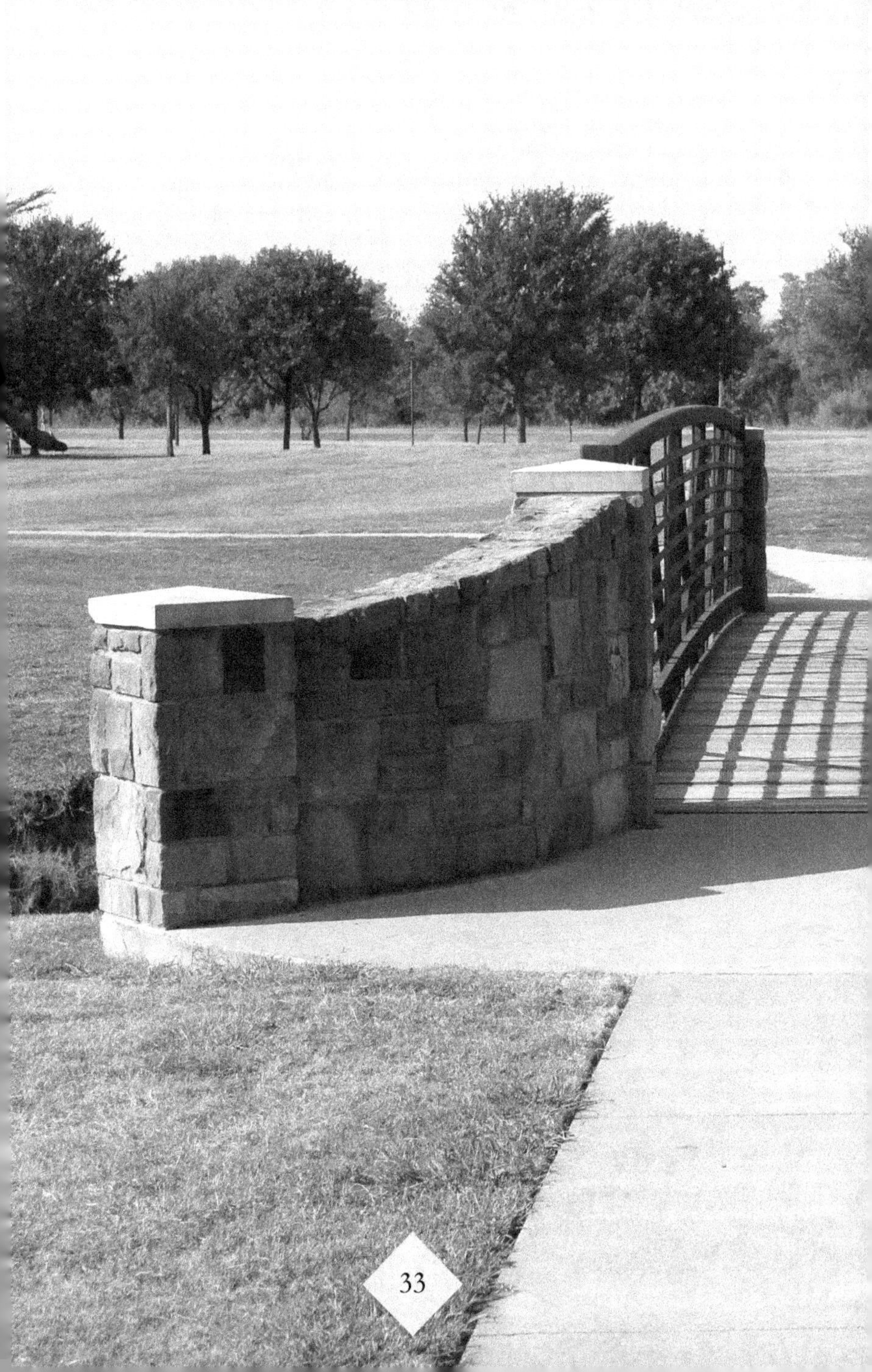

# Falling / Timber

As we get older, sometimes our brain thinks faster than how our body responds. When you are very tall, and with age, our knees begin to get stiff and feet don't lift as high off the ground as they should when we walk. One may not realize they are losing their balance until they fall.

Take standing, for instance. You may have gotten out of a chair and your butt is off the seat, but that does not mean you are actually standing and have your balance. One is on to the next task mentally, not realizing the task at hand is not complete. The result: timber! You have fallen back in your seat; across the bed; against the wall; or on the floor. "Did I do that?  What happened?" is the typical response.

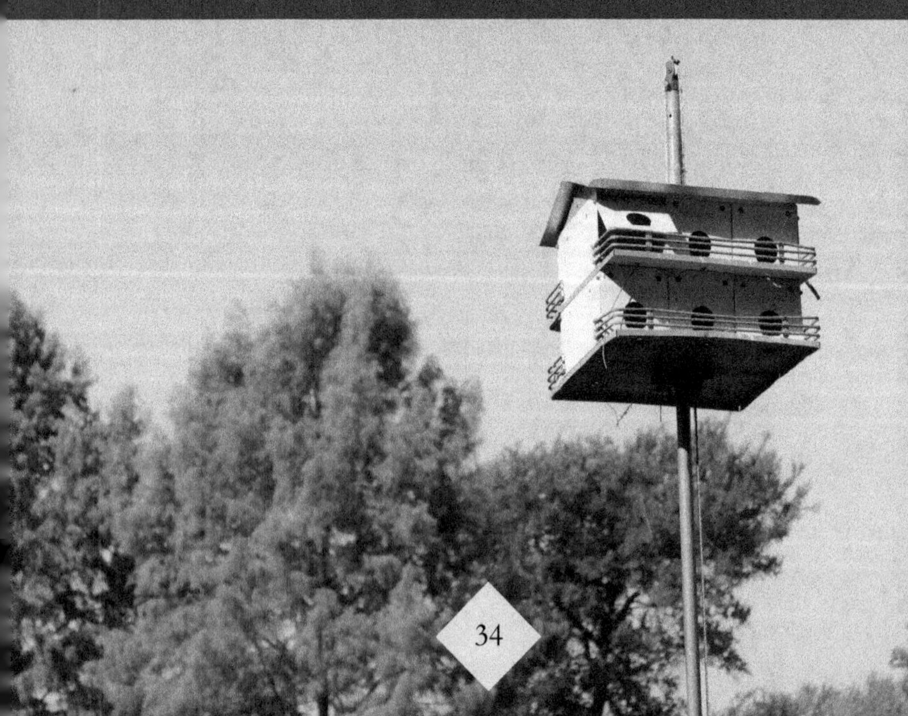

35

*Consider ways you can prevent your loved one from falling.*

# Get Help / Gather Information

Glean information and gather resources before you need it.   Online blogs and websites, healthcare professionals, local council on aging, library, community center, family, church and friends are all resources that can be lifelines.

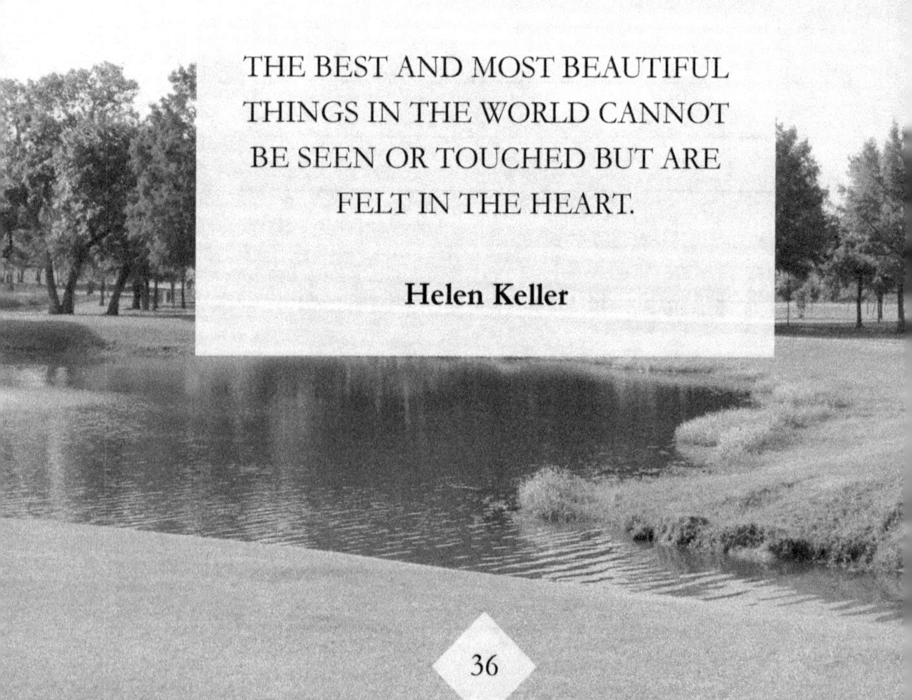

# Reflection / Action:

*Compile a list of resources.*

# Hide Pill Box Organizer

A new system was started of putting dad's meds in a pill box organizer which had a different section for each day of the week. This was to help dad know if he had taken his meds for the day. This day was different. It went as follows:

7:00 am      Dad got up. Checked mailbox. Took meds with juice. Went back to bed.

7:30 am      I checked on dad because he was in the kitchen again. He said he was finishing his juice, but I noticed his mouth was full and he could not talk. I decided to check the pill box and noticed Sunday and Monday meds had been taken.

8:00 am      I called home health care regarding implementation of the pill box they had recommended on an earlier visit, but dad had just taken two days of meds! Their recommendation to me was to: Go to the ER since high blood pressure meds could bring his pressure too low.

8:45 am      Admitted to ER. Monitored for 3 hours during which he needed continuous adjustments to his pillow, bed, covers, and pants' belt; as well as, an endless supply of tissue to blow his nose! Lesson learned.

# Information / Know before you Go

Know who, what, when, where and how before you go. Children ask, "Are we there, yet?" But, the grey-haired ask, "Where are we going?" "Do you know how to get there?" "What time is the appointment?" "Why are we going?" "Who told you this? They didn't tell me."

Be prepared to answer questions and have proof of the need to go, i.e. appointment card, grocery list, brochure, directions. Have an extra copy to give your loved one to read and hold on to.

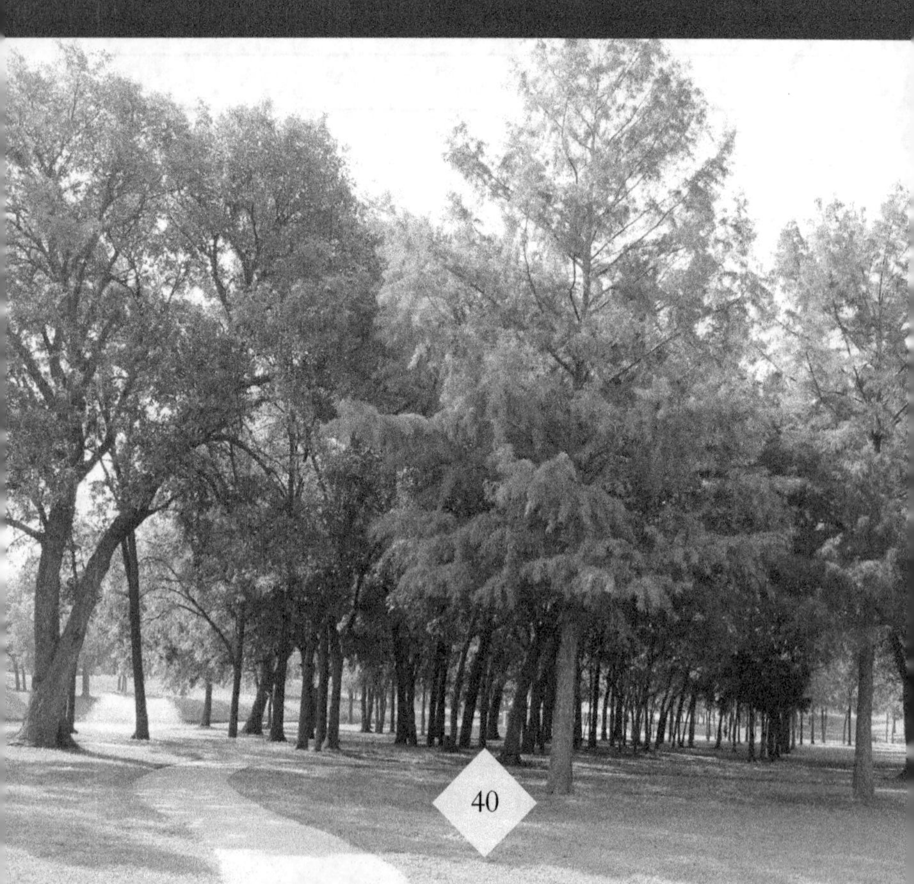

# Just Part of the Disease

After updating the doctor on the frequency of dad's "sundowning", he said he could give a prescription for agitation that would help him sleep.

Dad interjected, "Wait a minute!  [I] don't want anything to make me permanently sleep!"

We declined the additional meds.  Before we left, the doctor looked at me and said, "Hang on in there.  It is only going to get worse!"

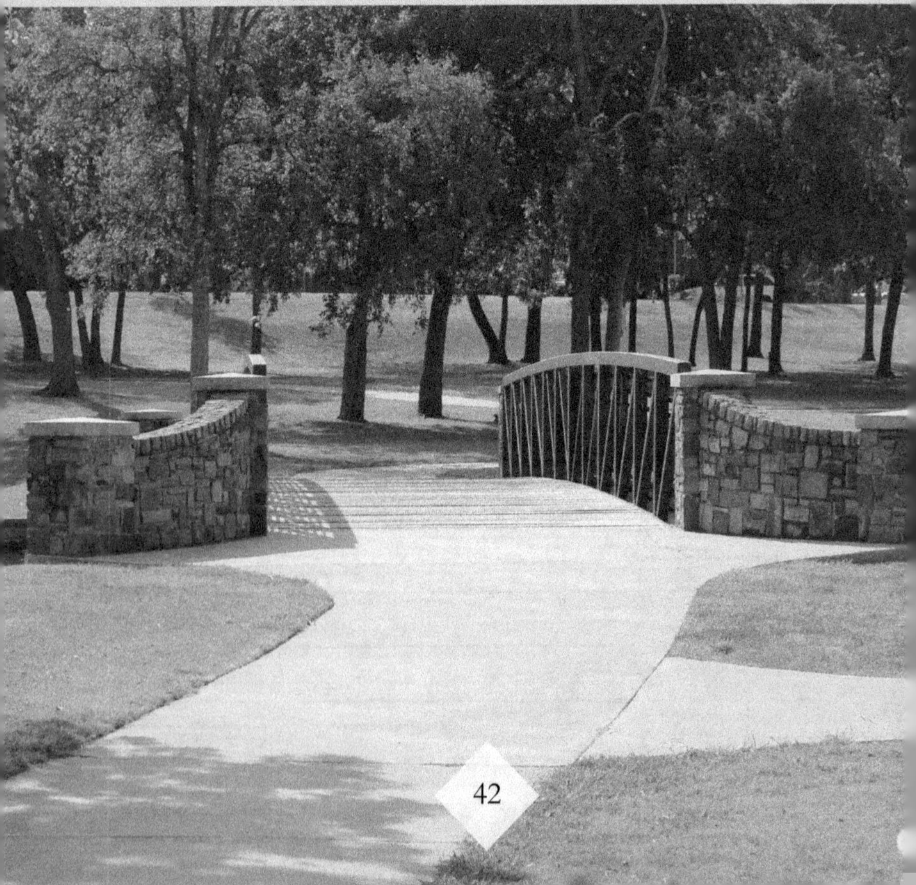

# Reflection / Action:

# Keep It Simple

» Options
» Activities
» Conversations
» Tasks
» Selections

Providing simple options and seeking your loved ones input on activities, conversations, tasks and selections helps their decision-making process, gives them a sense of control, and reduces frustrations.

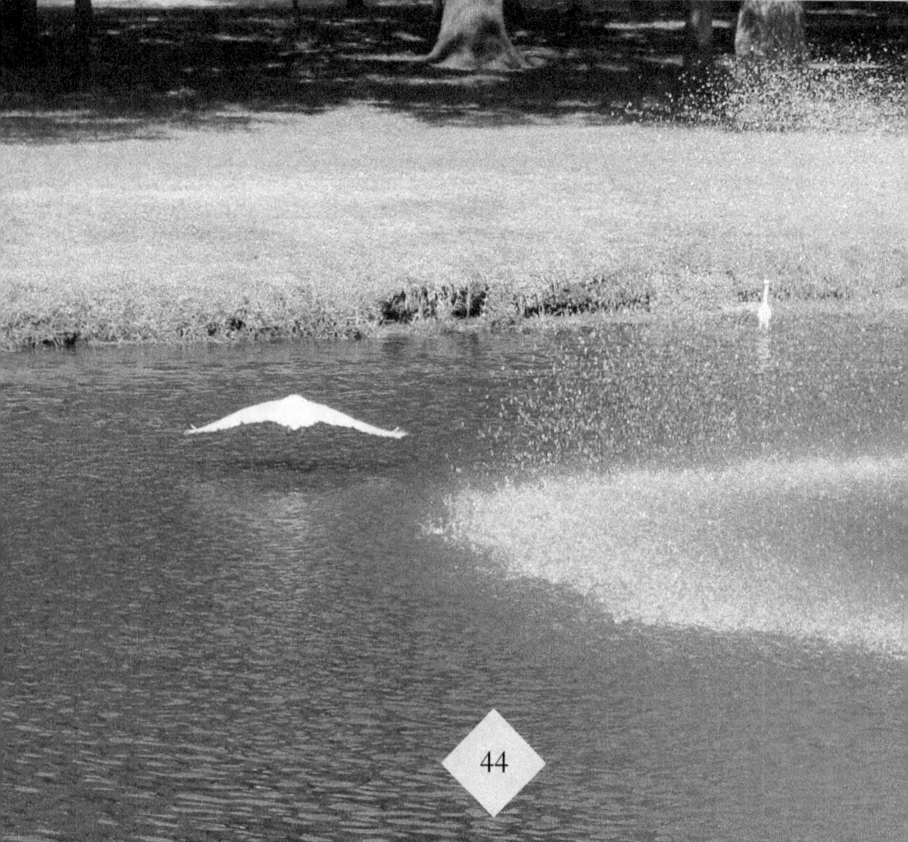

# Laugh / Love

Find moments to be light hearted and laugh at yourself and with your loved one.  Turn off the news and turn on something comical from the 1950's or the classic-tv era.

Turn the serious or do the mundane in love.  Look for ways to make it better and before you know it, it will turn into a moment of joy.

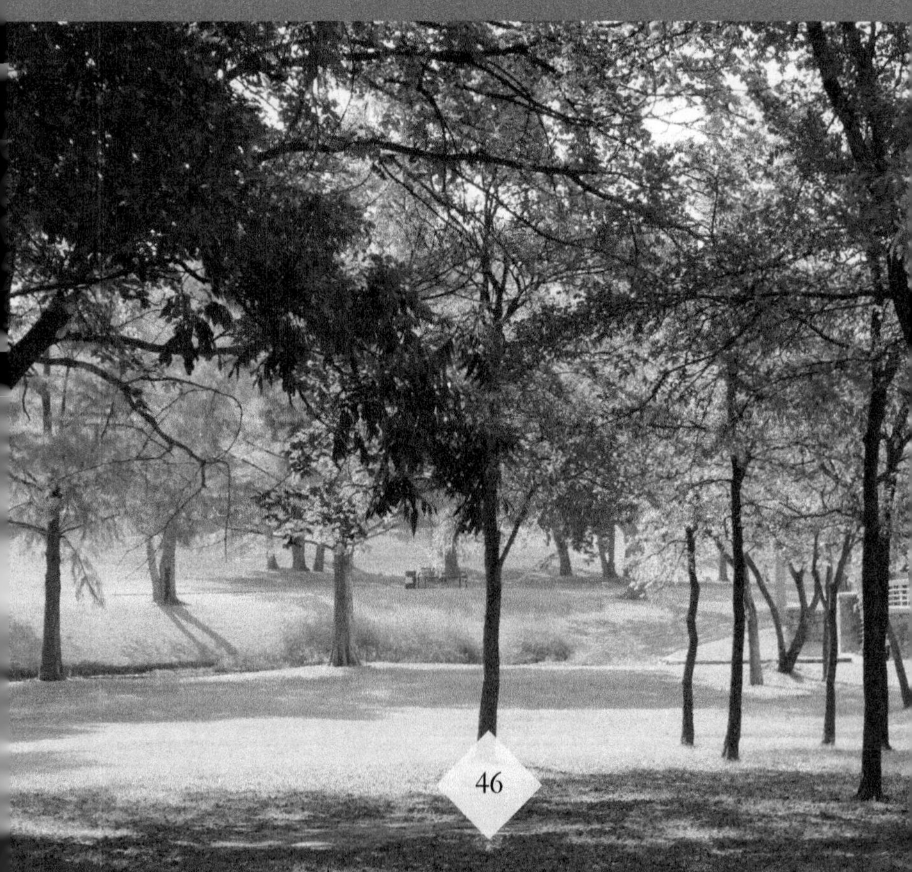

# Reflection / Action:

*Consider ways to have moments of laughter.*

# Make It a Great Day

You cannot change people, but you can change your attitude and outlook.

Make time for you. When things get stressful, take a moment to breathe, relax and rejuvenate. You may need to go to the other end of the house, close the door and scream.

Draw upon spiritual strength from a daily devotional, music or an inspirational program.

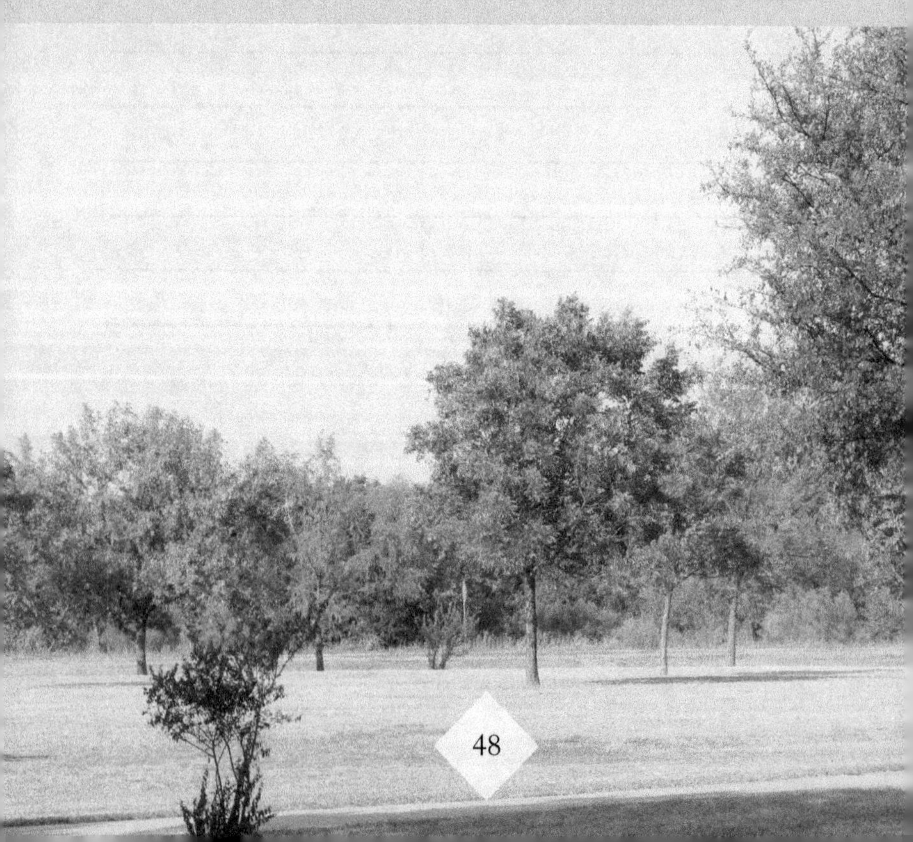

# Reflection / Action:

49

*Consider ways to have moments of laughter.*

# Noise

Be aware of sensitivity to noise, including:

» A/C or heater, blenders, microwave, washing machine, vent, or other noisy household equipment.
» Loud conversations or conversations involving more than two people may seem like arguing.
» Car horns blowing outside or on television.
» Violence or troubling news or programs on TV.

All these things can cause a change in your loved ones behavior or a call to action.

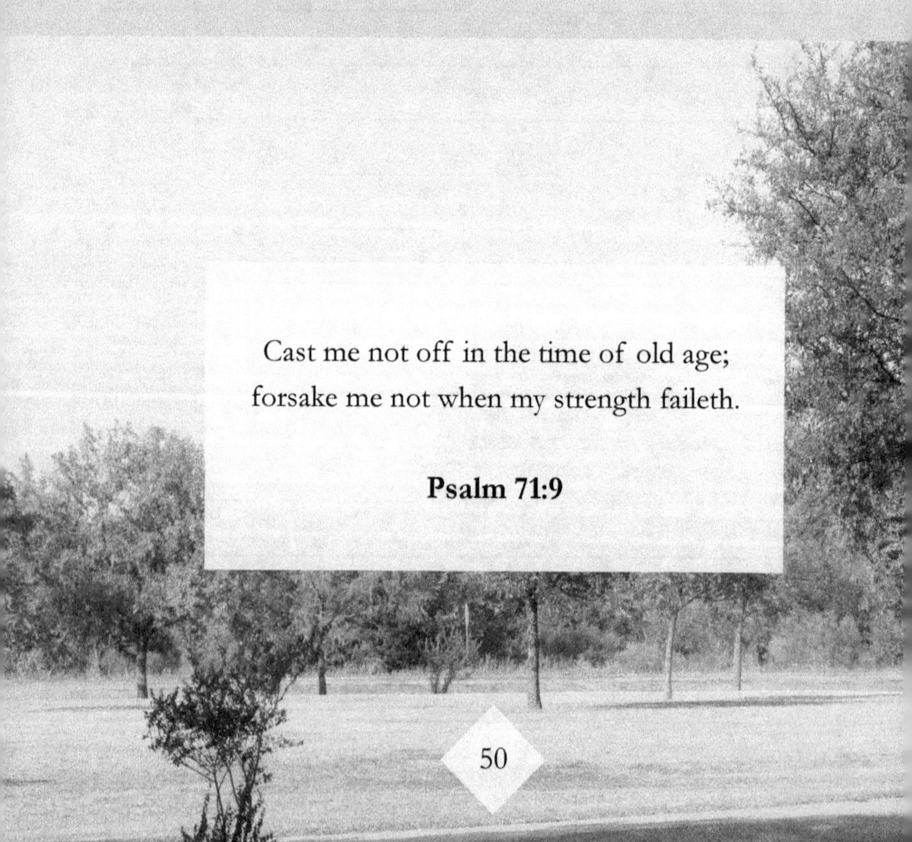

# Reflection / Action:

*Note behavioral changes that might be a result to loud noise.*

# Organizing Things

Dad started organizing his wallet.  He showed me everything in his brown leather, weathered, rubber band held wallet and said I needed to know the information.  He also started organizing the different cookies on the table and the baggies in the kitchen.

Constant rearranging things may seem like mindless work, but it gives a sense of productivity and accomplishment.  Don't be annoyed by busy work.

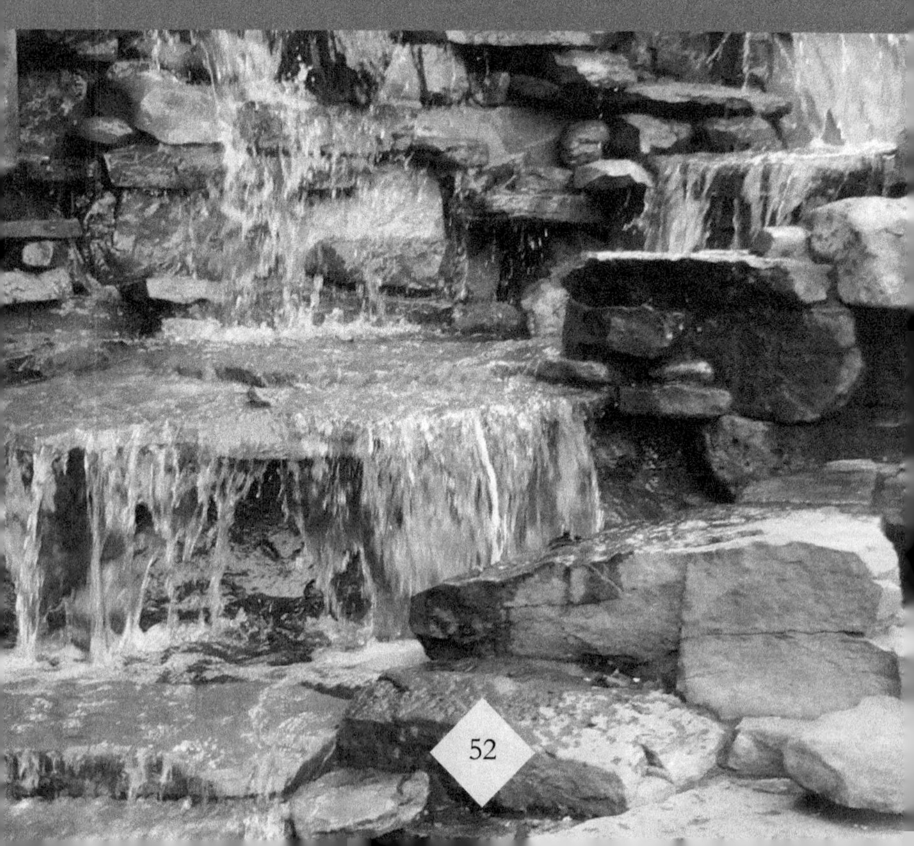

53

# Pictures

Large 8 ½ x 11 pictures are on the wall in dad's bedroom and den with labels to identify who is in the picture.
"Who is the little lady… the shortest one?"

"That's a big guy…need to get out of his way…his wife doesn't have a chance…she's probably holding her own…she has a family and is holding on to the Lord."

Regarding his formal Navy picture on the coffee table, dad said the photographer told him to take his cap off his head and put it on like it is shown in the picture – further back on his head.  It gives a better view of his facial features.

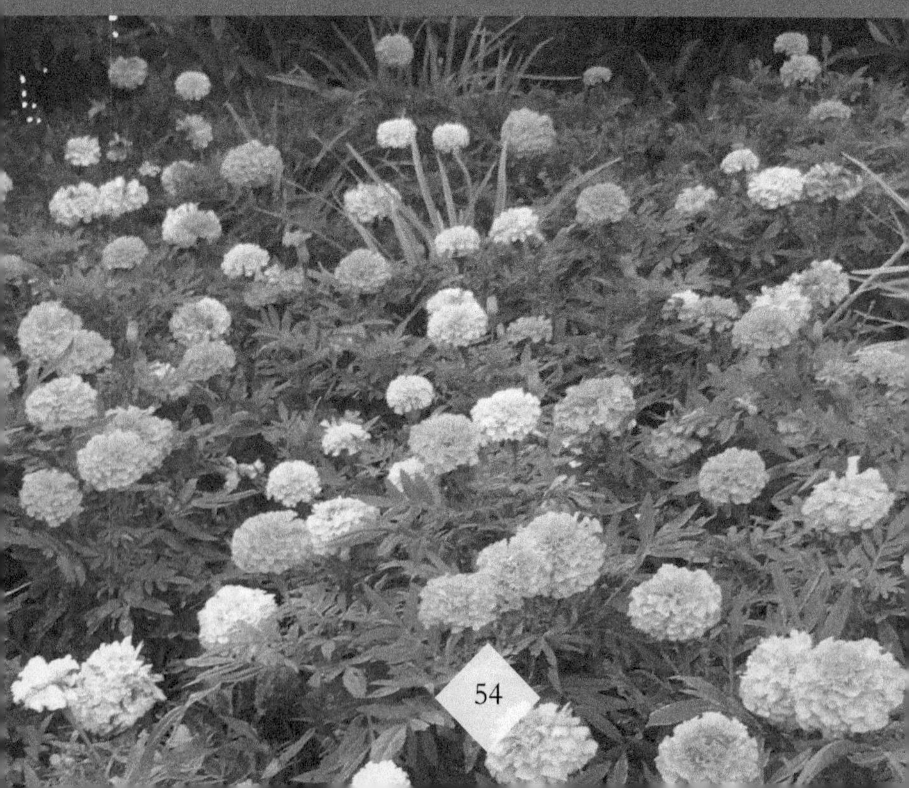

# Reflection / Action:

55

*Consider enlarging and captioning pictures to help stimulate memories.*

# Plan of Action

Part of being 'prepared before you go' is to have a plan of action when your loved one needs to go to the restroom. Have different routes in mind that have restaurants, gas stations or public buildings with easy access to restrooms.

Even when you get to your destination, ask if they need to go beforehand. Likewise, before leaving ask if they need to go again. Mentally, be prepared to take them before, during, after and in-route. Anticipate and be prepared.

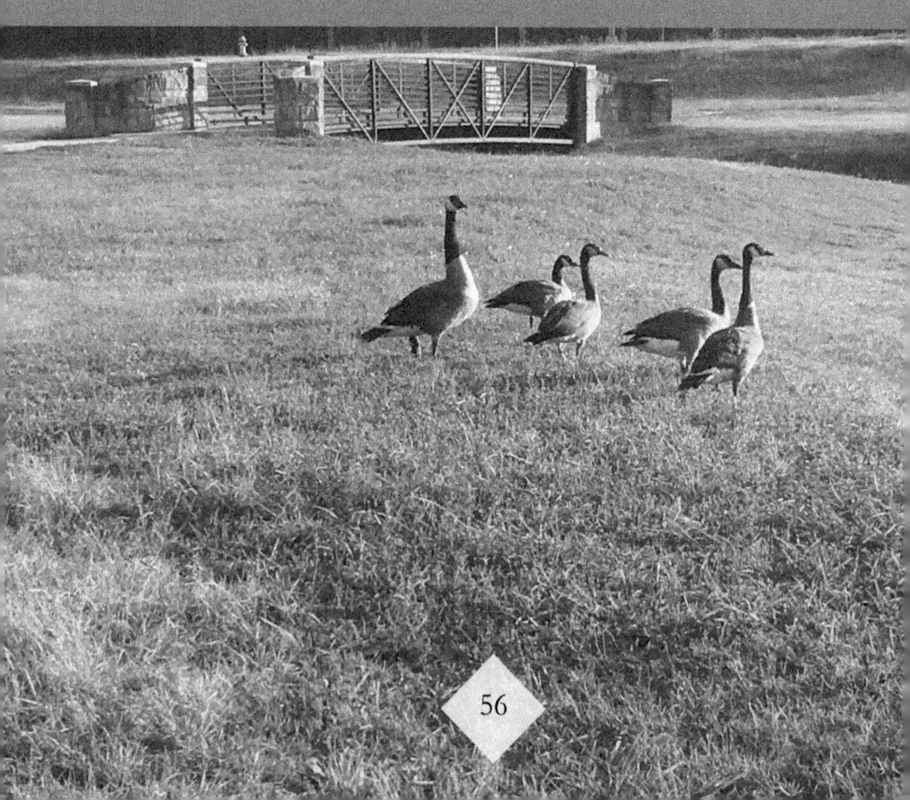

# Reflection | Action:

*List better ways you can be prepared for bathroom emergencies.*

# Quiet Time

You and your loved one should not always be busy.  Enjoy quiet time.

Respect your loved one's time alone when they may be reflecting or just want to move at their own pace.

Use your quiet time to journal and reflect.  It is amazing what you hear when you slow down and be still.

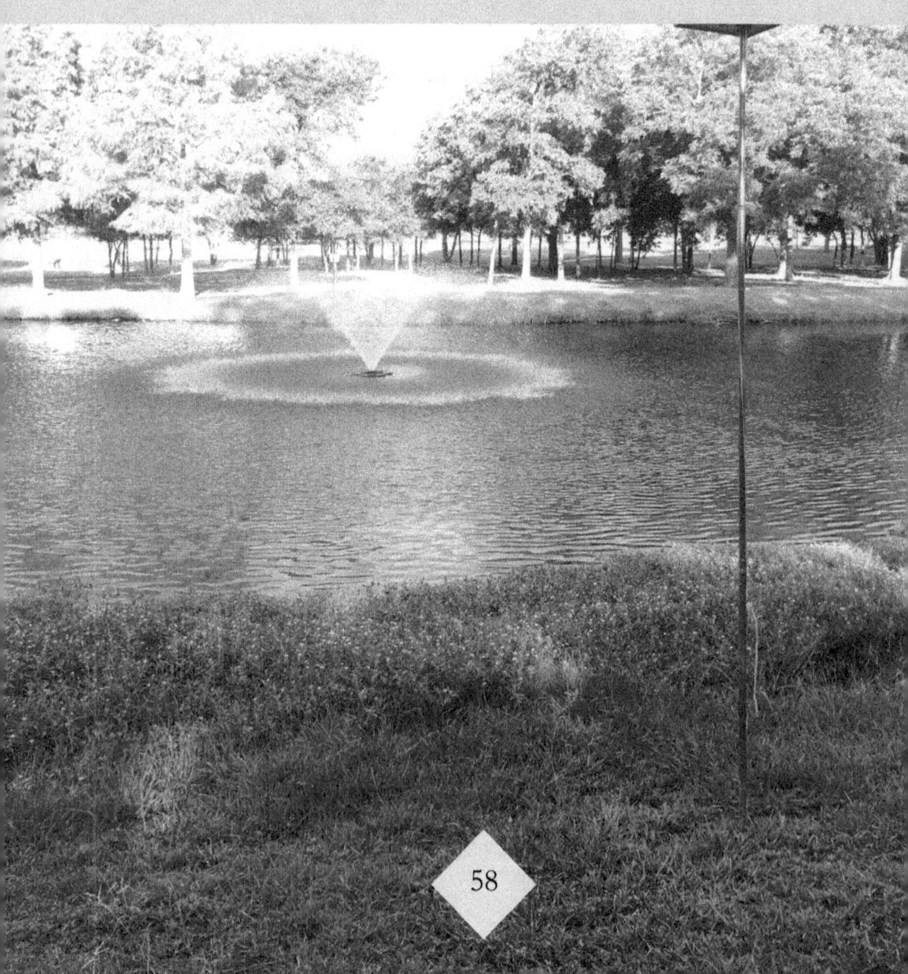

## Reflection / Action:

59

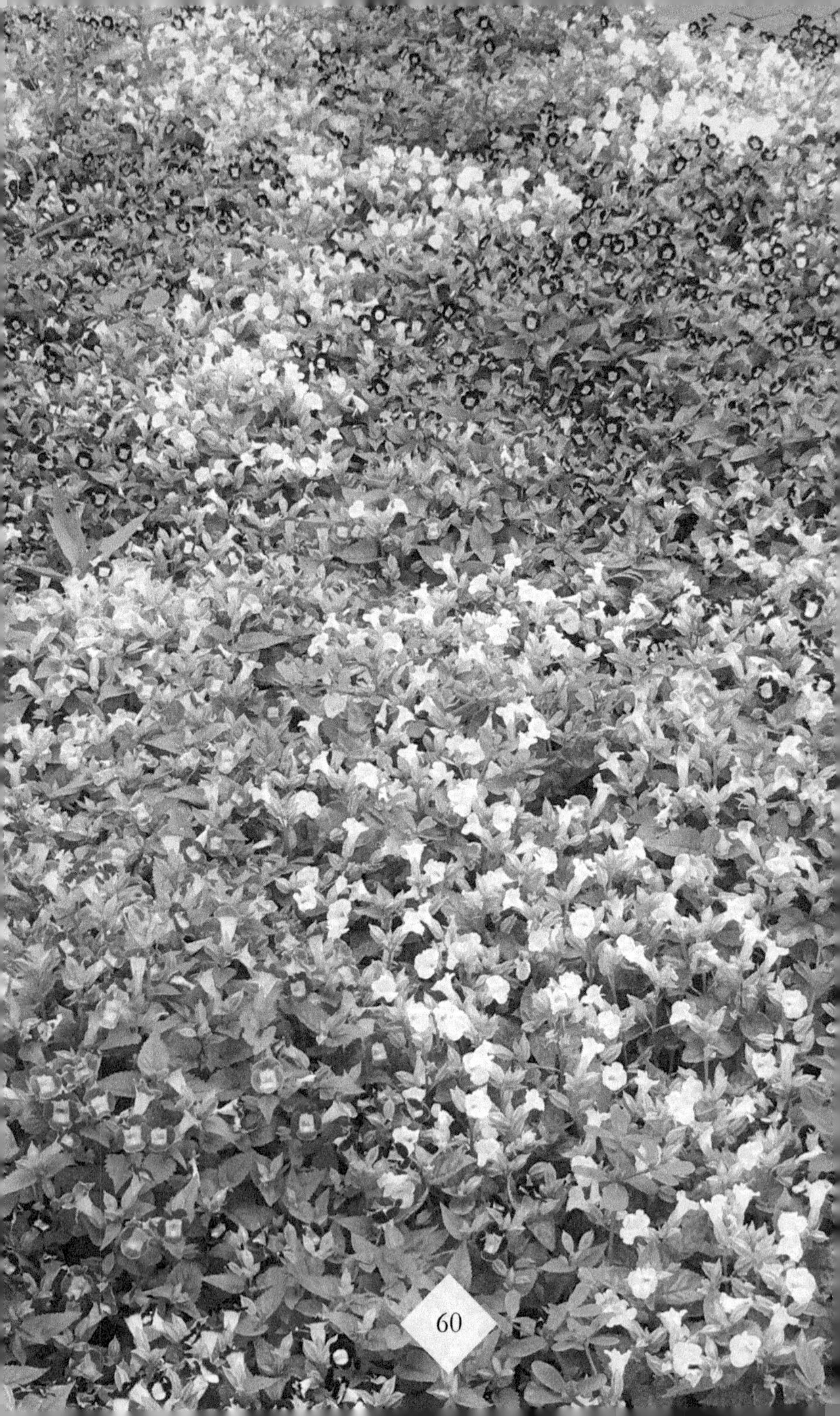
60

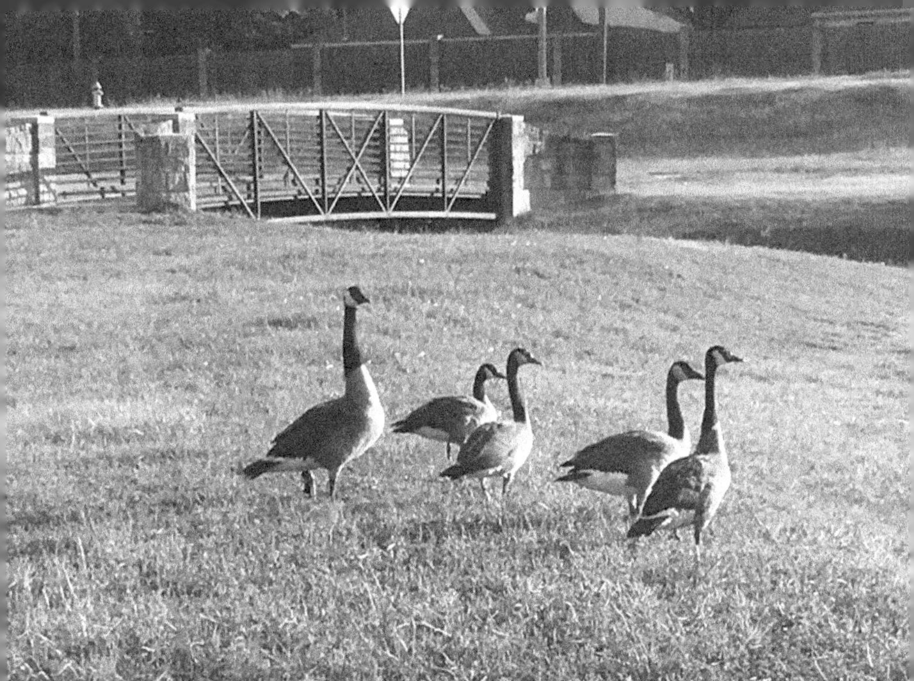

# Rhythm

When speaking or talking to loved ones, be on their eye level. If they are seated, then sit down. Mirror their tone and voice. Flow with their rhythm. Fast and loud talking or movement can make them anxious.

Follow their pace. Reduce background noises and distractions when communicating.

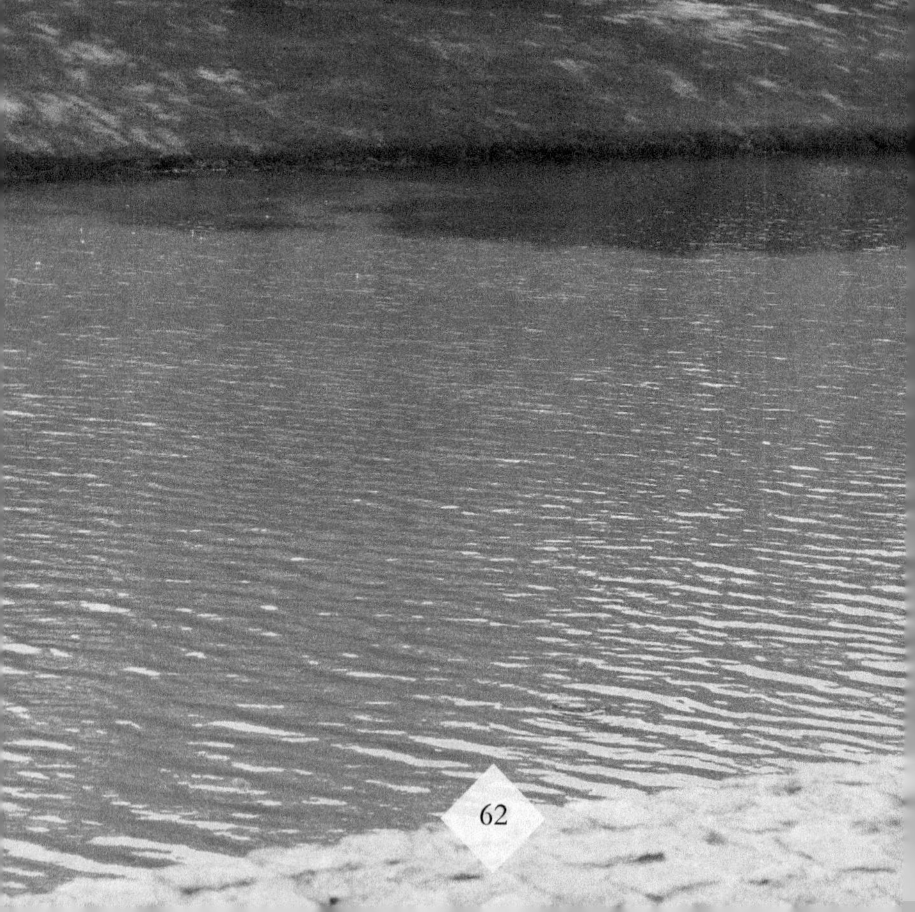

## Reflection / Action:

# Support Groups

Structured support groups sponsored by retirement facilities provide a wide spectrum of resources, such as:

**Nutrition and Dementia**
**Separation Anxiety**
**Caregiver Stress**
**Techniques for Communicating**
**Balance Falls and Dementia**
**Grief and the Loss of Loved One**
**Sleep and the Dementia Patient**
**Benefits of Music Therapy**
**Estate Planning/Elder Care**
**Hospice and Dementia**
**Getting Financially Prepared for Dementia**
**Helping You and Your Loved One with**
**Dementia Maintain Quality of Life**
**Validation Theory Techniques**

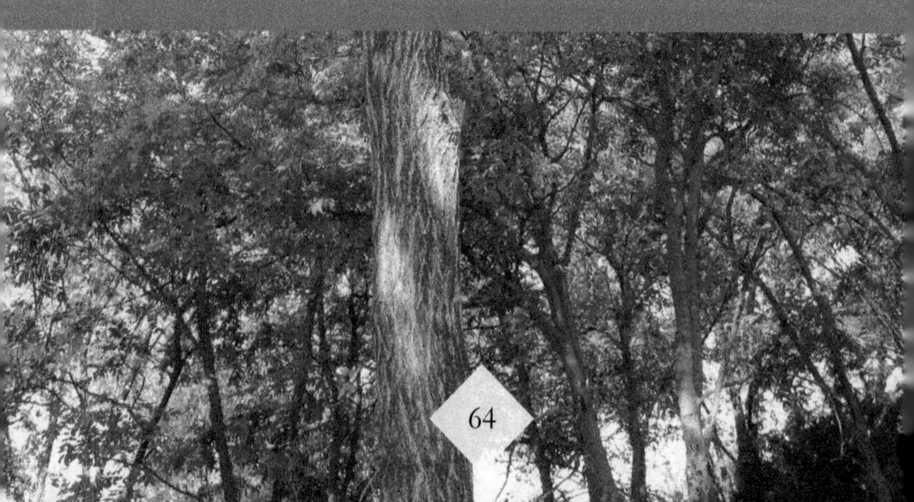

# Reflection / Action:

*List other resources in your local area.*

# Timing is Everything

Reduce stress by planning appointments in the mornings, early afternoons or the best time of day for your loved one.

Appointments should be made to minimize wait time.  It also helps to schedule on days that do not interfere with deliveries or other home care services.

If your loved one had a bad night and did not get much rest prior to an appointment, it might be wise to reschedule in order to reduce their anxiety and level of frustration.

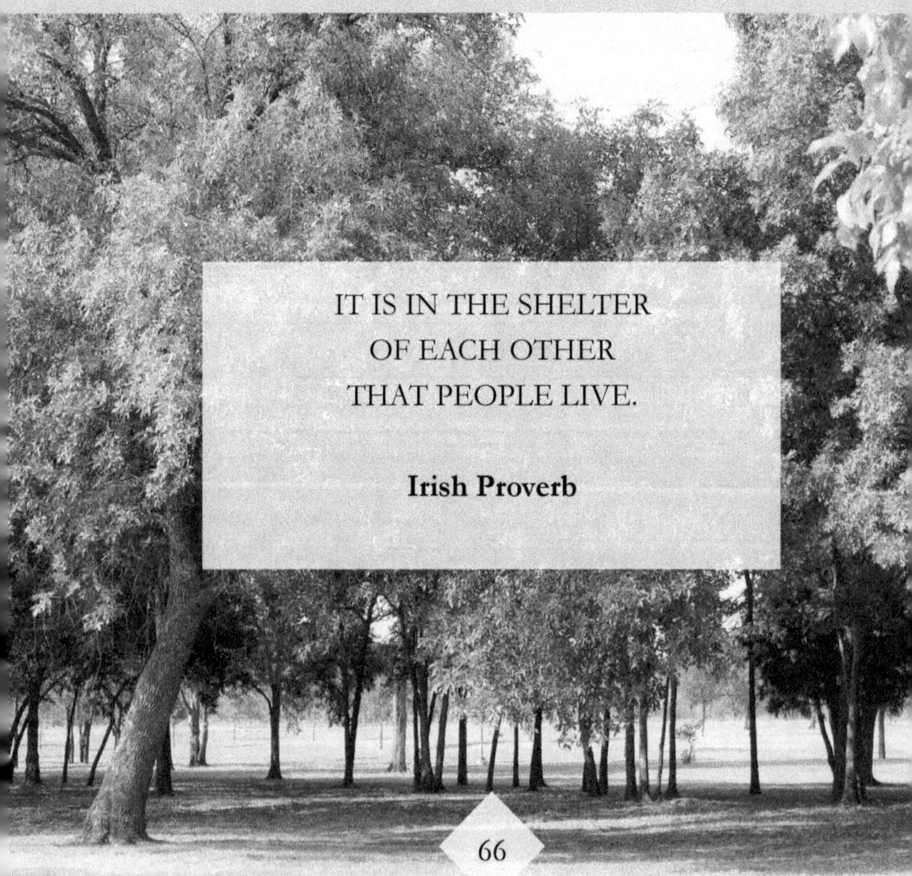

# Reflection | Action:

*What is the best day of the week and time of the day to schedule an appointment for your loved one?*

# Understand Their Needs

Always understand your loved ones needs and point of view. Sometimes unusual behavior represents a change in needs that has not been or can not be articulated. A physical or medical need might be expressed in an emotional behavior.

Many times, caregivers can become task-oriented and may not be sensitive to emotional needs and/or root-cause behavior.

Sometimes you just need to sit with them and be close at hand.

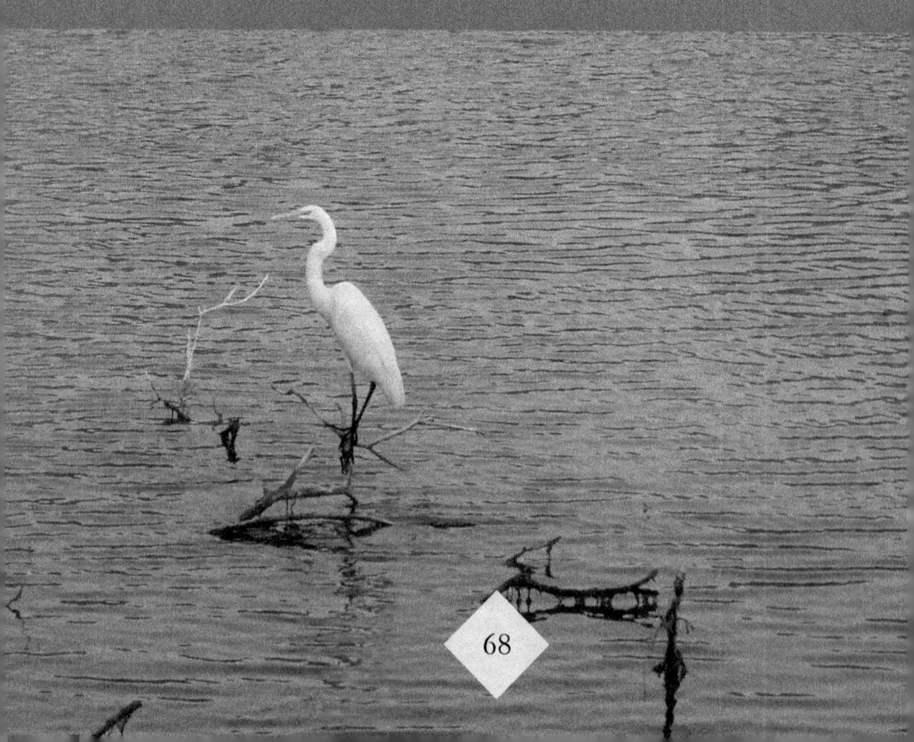

# Reflection / Action:

*Note changes in behavior that might be an indication of a need.*

# Verify

Verify, ask questions, and double check medications, the need for medical procedures, insurance coverage, qualifications for services and programs, financial statements, daily living expenses and fees.

> » Don't assume anything.
> » Get information.
> » Check the facts.
> » Obtain it in writing.
> » Document everything and keep good notes.

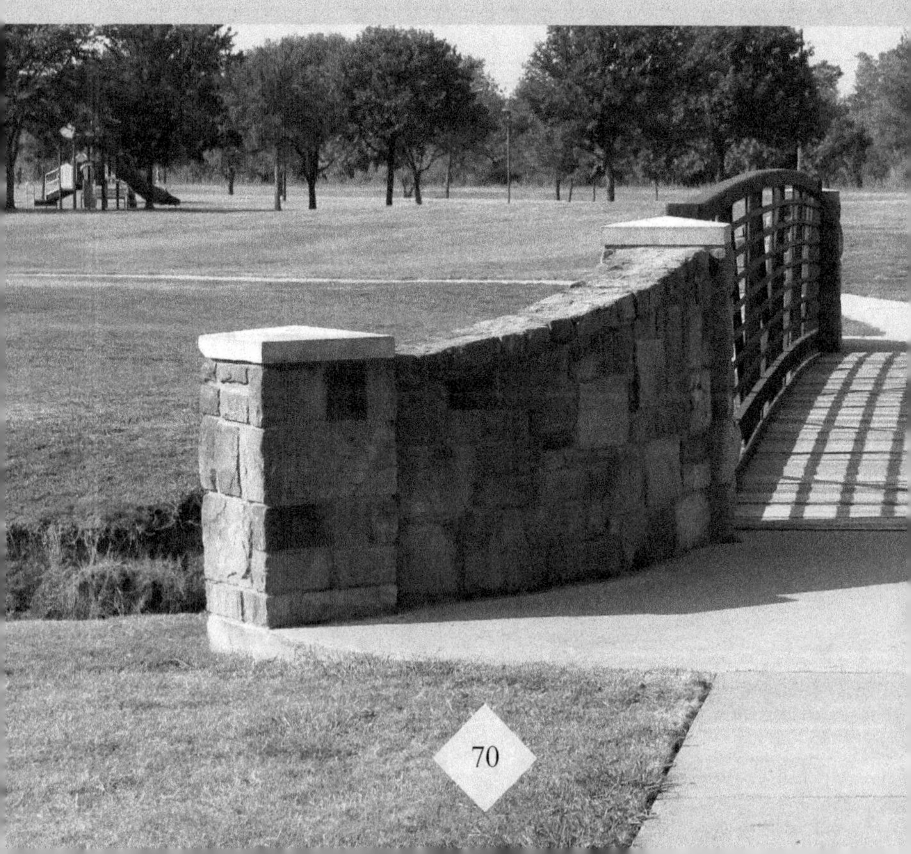

# Reflection / Action:

*Make a to-do list of services, resources and / or bills to follow-up on.*

# Wandering

It's 11:30 p.m. and dad just walked down the hall with his jeans, tennis shoes and housecoat on, carrying his urinal, tissue and car keys in hand.  Later, it was discovered he had his nose spray and clippers in this coat pocket.  I asked if he was going somewhere?  He proceeded to go out the side door to the car.

Even though it was night outside, he did not realize that because the carport light was on.  While he was fidgeting with the keys, I ran and checked his bedroom.  Yep, the sheets needed to be changed! Once the bed linen was changed, he was advised and he came on in the house.

Wandering has a purpose.

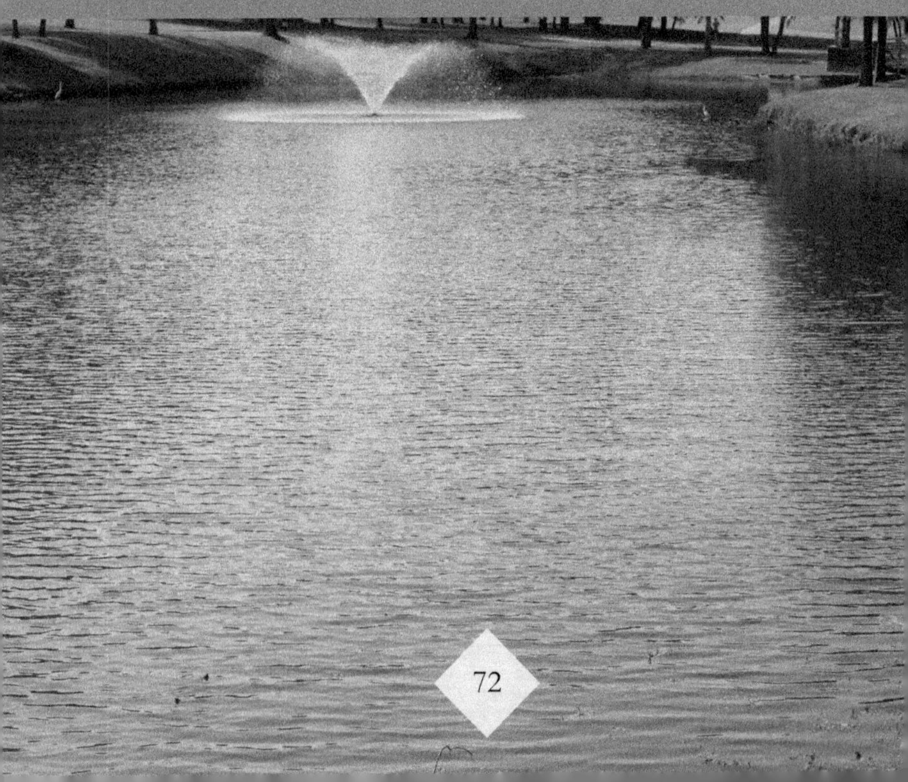

*Consider unusual behavior your loved one may have in response to an unspoken issue.*

# White Board / Reminder Notes / Stickers

A good way to aid in memory is to have a reminder board and to leave large notes.

Daily the white board on the refrigerator is updated with the day of the week and the date.  In addition, it is a good place to put medical appointments, scheduled visits and other reminders.

Additional reminders can be written in markers on a large piece of paper and placed by the bed, on the table and by the door.

Lastly, my sister made labels and placed them on items, as reminders.

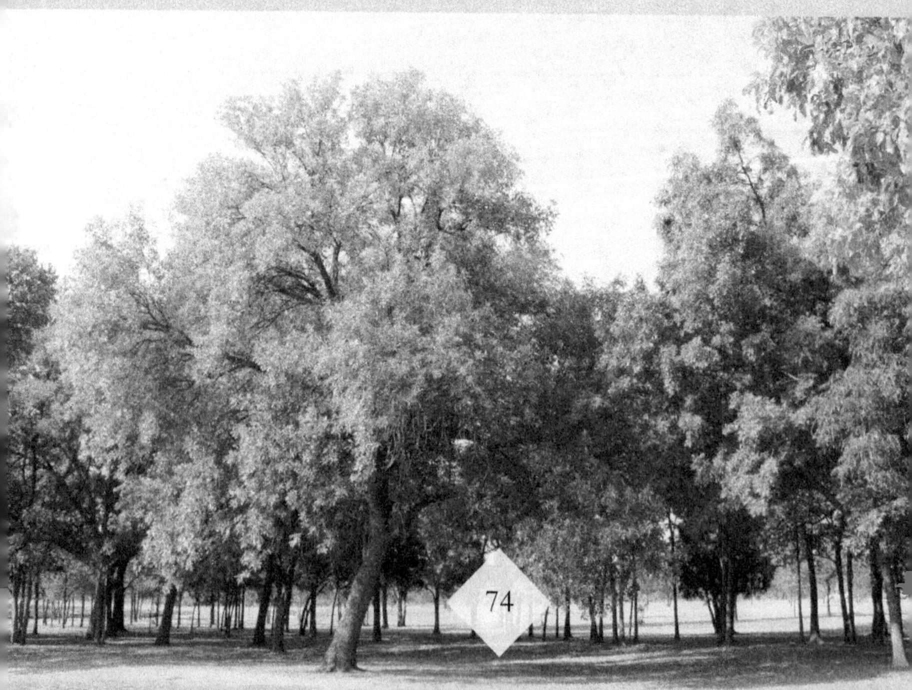

# eXamine / eXercise Rights

Examine old contracts and policies.  Asks for updates, revisions and/or special rates.

Have health care providers update medical privacy authorizations.  Have appropriate conversations regarding medical wishes and living wills.

Obtain legal authority, power of attorney (POA), etc. to act on behalf of your love one and exercise their rights.

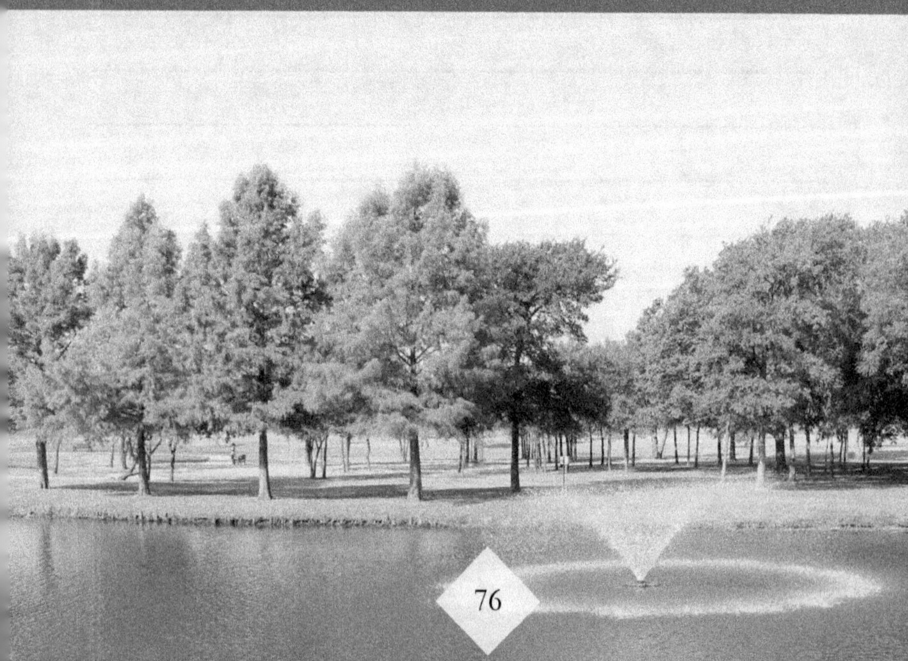

# Reflection / Action:

*List service providers to be contacted and other things to follow through on.*

# You are the Advocate

Use your voice and be the advocate for your loved one.

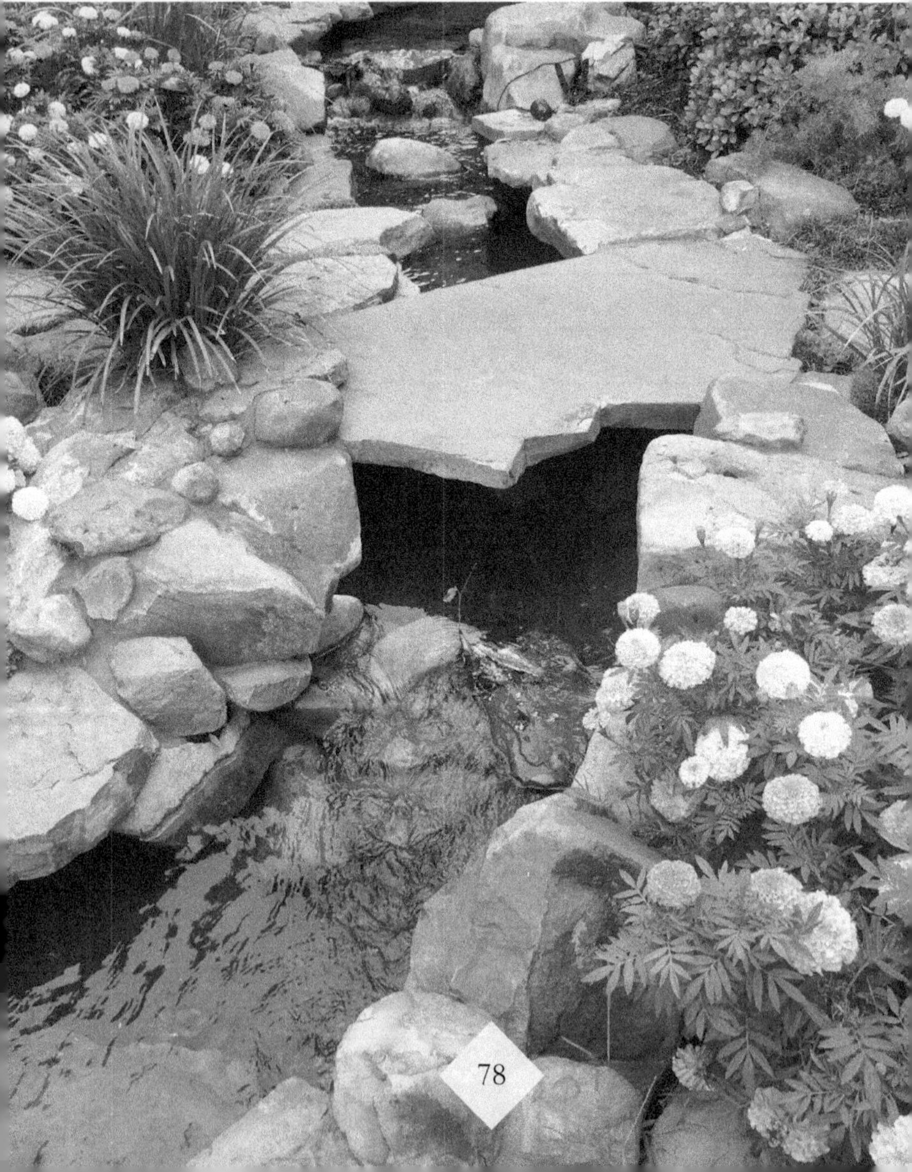

# *Reflection | Action:*

*List ways you can speak up and out on behalf of your loved one.*

# Zoom IN

Zoom in on past and current conversations where your love one has expressed a need or action that has not been completed.

Don't blow them off as 'just talking'.  Focus on the outstanding business that they need your help addressing or completing.

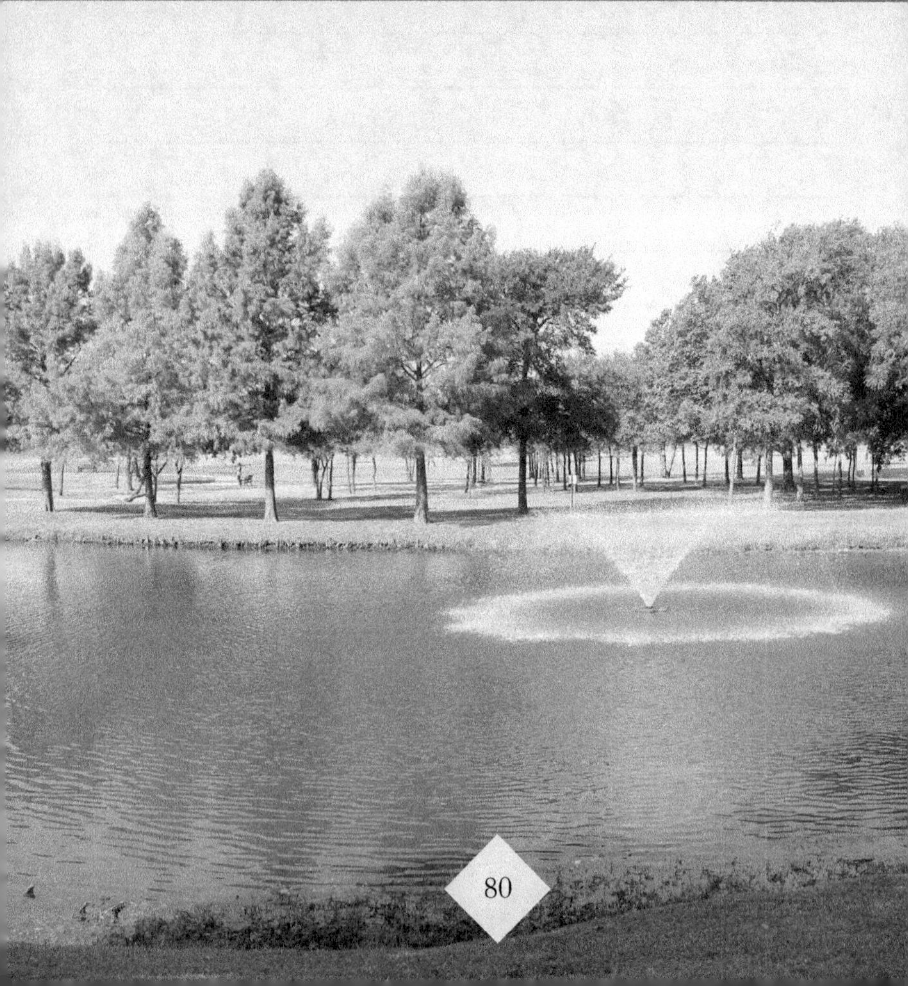

# Reflection / Action:

*Record any outstanding wishes or requests made by your loved one.*

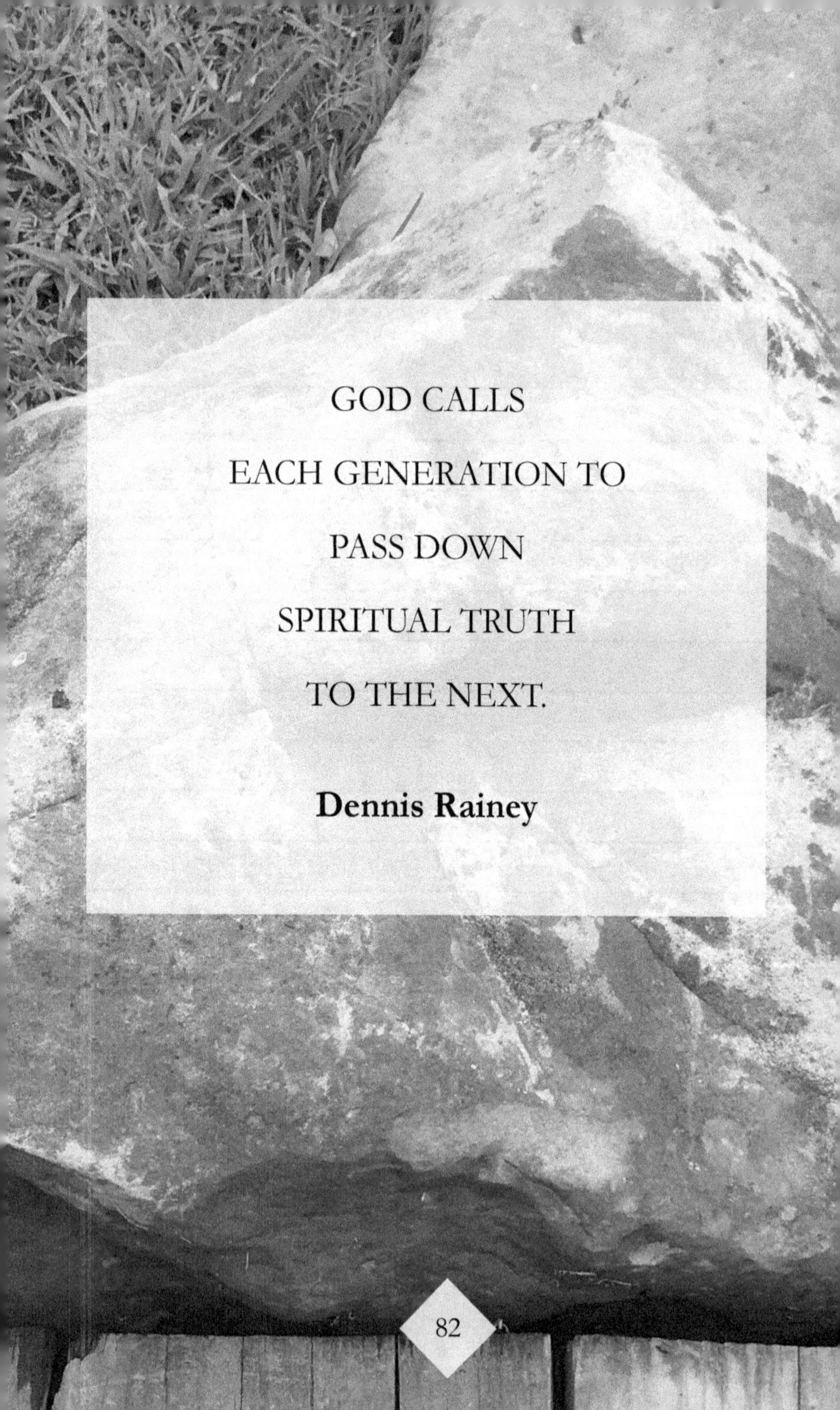

GOD CALLS
EACH GENERATION TO
PASS DOWN
SPIRITUAL TRUTH
TO THE NEXT.

Dennis Rainey

# References

Brackey, Jolene. (2007).  Creating Moments of Joy for the Person with Alzheimer's or Dementia.  Enhanced Moments.

Feil, Naomi. (2002).  The Validation Breakthrough, Simple Techniques for Communicating with People with "Alzheimer's-Type Dementia?" Baltimore, MD: Health Professionals Press.

Gibbs, Terri (ed.). (2000).   A Father's Legacy. Your Life Story in Your Own Words. Nashville, TN: J. Countryman.

(2015) Alzheimer's Disease Facts and Figures, Alzheimer's Association.

# ABOUT THE AUTHOR

Verna R. Jacobs is the oldest child of Bunyan Jacobs, Jr. Having the privilege to know and grow up with many fathers and all four of her grandparents, Verna knows first-hand the depth and levels of wisdom, knowledge, and understanding that can be gleaned from elders. These principles have afforded her with a rich heritage which has been the driving force in creating this project.

It is Verna's desire that this book show love, honor and respect to her father, as well as, provide humor, inspiration and encouragement for other caregivers, family and friends who have loved ones with dementia. Enjoy the journey! Verna encourages others to document their stories to extend their legacies and produce a gift that keeps on giving.

For more information, please visit alifewithalz.com.

# COMING IN FALL 2017

## by
## Verna Jacobs

A Life with Alzheimer's:
A Digest of Dad's ALZs
(Anecdotes, Laughs, Zingers and Stories)

~

A Life with Alzheimer's:
A Memoir and Reflections of a Dad and a Daughter

~

**SUBSCRIBE ONLINE FOR AUTHOR UPDATES:**
www.alifewithalz.com

# OTHER BOOKS
# BY
# THIS AUTHOR

When I Look Back:
A Memoir of Alene Delaney Simmons
Available on Amazon

9 781977 754486